CORONARY HEART DISEASE

A GUIDE *to* DIAGNOSIS *and* TREATMENT

SECOND EDITION

BARRY M. COHEN, M.D. • BOBBIE HASSELBRING

Addicus Books
Omaha, Nebraska

An Addicus Nonfiction Book

Second Edition   ISBN 978-1-886039-83-4

Cover design by George Foster
Illustrations by Jack Kusler
Interior design by Concord Editorial and Design

This book is not intended to serve as a substitute for a physician, nor do the authors intend to offer medical advice contrary to that of an attending physician.

Library of Congress Cataloging-in-Publication Data

Cohen, Barry M.
  Coronary heart disease: a guide to diagnosis and treatment /
Barry M. Cohen, Bobbie Hasselbring. -- 2nd ed.
      p. cm.
  Includes index.
  1. Coronary heart disease -- Popular works. I. Hasselbring,
Bobbie, 1951– II. Title.
  RC685.C6C58 2007
  616.1'23—dc22

2006103098

Addicus Books
P.O. Box 45327
Omaha, Nebraska 68145
www.AddicusBooks.com

Printed in the United States of America
10 9 8 7 6 5 4 3 2 1

To my parents,
Elaine and Gerry Cohen

Contents

Foreword

More people are affected by atherosclerosis, commonly referred to as "hardening of the arteries," than by any other single disorder. On the nightly news we hear quite a lot about the effects of atherosclerosis—stroke, loss of limbs, heart attack, and death. Our friends and family recall those who have been touched by or even died from atherosclerosis. Though you may worry more about cancer, you *should* be more concerned about heart disease, stroke, and leg artery disease.

Atherosclerosis doesn't affect just the heart, it affects the entire body. If you have a blockage in one artery, odds are that you have blockages in other arteries elsewhere in the body. For instance, if you have leg artery blockage, there is a 50/50 chance that you also have heart artery blockage. If you have heart artery blockage, there is a 30 percent chance that you have significant blockage of the artery that brings blood to the brain. This is why early diagnosis and aggressive prevention are the keys to surviving atherosclerosis and coronary heart disease (CHD).

This book is designed to help you understand what a heart attack is, how doctors can determine if you have heart artery blockage even if you don't have symptoms, and what treatments are available. *Coronary Heart Disease: A Guide to Diagnosis and Treatment* will help you understand why smoking is so bad for you and how lowering your high cholesterol is an excellent method of reducing your risk of heart attack and death from CHD.

This book gives you valuable and up-to-date information, your most powerful weapon against atherosclerosis and heart disease. I urge you to read every page—for your good health and for your heart's good health.

> — Michael R. Jaff, D.O.
> Director, Vascular Medicine
> Massachusetts General Hospital,
> Assistant Professor of Medicine
> Harvard Medical School
> Boston, Massachusetts

Acknowledgments

It's not the destination. It's the journey. This book has been a wonderful journey, which would not have been possible without the invaluable assistance and insights from my colleagues, family, and friends.

From the Gagnon Heart Hospital at Overlook and Morristown in New Jersey, I would like to thank Drs. Frank Smart and Grant Parr; Dr. John Brown III, chief of cardiothoracic surgery, and his associates, Drs. Alejandro Rodriguez, Christopher Magovern, and James Slater; Emily Rowan, LCSW, and Janette Carlucci of the Cardiac Integrative Medicine Department; and Stanley Ort, RVT, RDCS, director of noninvasive services, who were invaluable resources. I also thank my cardiology colleagues from the Associates in Cardiovascular Disease (Springfield, Summit, and New Providence, NJ), Dr. Steven Rosenthal and the late Dr. Stephen Fischl. I am grateful for my outstanding hospital and office support team, including administrators, physician assistants, nurse practitioners, nurses, technologists, medical assistants, secretaries, and custodial personnel (you all know who you are).

Kathy Cohen, RD, of the Toronto Western Hospital was

exceptionally helpful sharing her perspectives and expertise in nutrition.

In addition, I am deeply indebted to my former professors, Drs. Valentin Fuster and Jose Meller, and the faculty at the Mount Sinai Medical Center in New York; Drs. Maurice Buchbinder and L. Kirk Peterson from the University of California San Diego Medical Center; Drs. Harold Frank and Irwin Labin, Mr. Herbert Bernard and the late Dr. Seymour Cohen for their wisdom, expertise, and inspiration.

I would also like to thank my publisher, Rod Colvin of Addicus Books, for his outstanding editing skills and for his clear vision for this book. Without Rod, this project would not be a reality. I also thank Jack Kusler for his work on the illustrations.

I am deeply appreciative of my parents, Elaine and Gerry Cohen, for their love, guidance, and encouragement throughout my studies and medical career. My parents have also been role models to me; their sixty years of marriage is a testament to their heart healthy lifestyle. I thank Ellen and Sam Weinstock for their assistance and advice. I am most grateful to my wife Jill and our children—Sara, Brett, and Chloe—for their love, encouragement, and endless support.

Finally, I'd like to thank my many patients and their families who have given me a great sense of professional and personal fulfillment as well as a heightened commitment to humanity each and every day.

—Barry M. Cohen, M.D.

Introduction

Coronary heart disease (CHD) is the number one killer in North America. Although there isn't a cure yet, there are many excellent treatments available to control symptoms and help people live long and healthy lives. We now have the technology to detect CHD early, even before you have symptoms, which may help decrease your risk of a heart attack. We wrote this book to give you the latest and best information about CHD so you can survive and even thrive despite it.

The goal of this book is to empower you with information about CHD. It can help you understand what CHD is, how to prevent it, how to find out if you have it, and finally, how best to treat it. By educating you about the risk factors for CHD, we hope to help you and your loved ones lower the risk for heart attack, stroke, and death. By informing you about the latest diagnostic and treatment techniques for people with early or advanced CHD, you, with your doctor, can make the best decisions to treat your disease. By giving you sound advice about lifestyle changes and medications, we give you the tools to stop—and possibly even reverse—your CHD.

People with CHD—or any illness for that matter—do best when they have a solid partnership with their health-care team. The more informed you are, the better this team can work for you. After reading this book, it is our hope that you will be a more informed partner in protecting your heart.

1 Understanding Coronary Heart Disease

"You have coronary heart disease." When your doctor says those words to you or to someone you love, it's frightening and confusing. You undoubtedly have dozens of questions: What is coronary heart disease? Why did I get it? Do I need medication? Will I need surgery? Do I need to change my lifestyle? Hopefully, this book will answer these questions and many more.

What Is Coronary Heart Disease?

Coronary heart disease (CHD), also called *coronary artery disease (CAD)* or *ischemic heart disease*, is a form of heart disease that's caused by narrowing of the coronary arteries that feed the heart. If you or someone you love has been diagnosed with CHD, it may help to know that you are not alone. In fact, CHD is the most common form of heart disease, affecting at least 12 million Americans. It is the single largest killer of both men and women in the United States, responsible for nearly a half million deaths each year, or about one out of every five deaths. CHD causes nearly all heart attacks (myocardial infarctions). Every twenty-nine seconds, an American suffers a coronary event, and every minute one of us will die from one. The American Heart Association estimates that this year alone, more than a million Americans will suffer from a new or recurrent coronary event, and nearly 40 percent of those will die from it.

Coronary heart disease isn't just an American problem. It is also very common in Europe and other Westernized countries. Diseases of the heart and circulation, such as heart attacks and strokes ("brain attacks"), kill more people worldwide than any other cause. The World Health Organization estimates that as many as 30 percent of all deaths are caused by heart and circulation diseases such as CHD.

The good news is that you don't have to become another CHD statistic. There is much you can do to reduce your risk of having a heart attack or dying from CHD. Sometimes just changing your lifestyle—following a heart-healthy diet, exercising regularly, and reducing the stress in your life—can prevent a heart attack or even reverse the narrowing in your arteries. There are a number of medications—and new ones being developed every day—that can help lower your heart attack risk. Surgical procedures such as angioplasty and stenting or bypass surgery can help compensate for blockages in your arteries and help keep your heart supplied with the blood it needs. By educating yourself about your treatment options with books such as this one and by working closely with your doctor, you and your doctor can choose the treatments that will best enable you to live a long and healthy life.

The Circulatory System

The first step in taking charge of your CHD is to learn all you can about the disease. To understand what CHD is and how it affects your heart, you need to understand a little about your heart and how it works.

Your *circulatory system*, also called your *cardiovascular system*, is made up of the heart, the lungs, and blood vessels called *arteries* and *veins*. This system carries blood, food, and oxygen to every cell in the body. It also carries waste products away from the cells and out of the body. (A *cell* is the building block of every tissue and organ in the body.) Think of your circulatory system as a busy highway system composed of massive freeways and large streets that feed into smaller and smaller streets, and finally into tiny lanes and alleyways. This system is made up entirely of one-way streets. In our imaginary highway system, cars, or in this case, blood, can flow in only *one* direction. The one-way streets called arteries and *arterioles* (small arteries) carry blood enriched with oxygen and nutrients away from the heart to the cells in the body. The one-way streets called veins and *venules* (small veins) carry blood loaded with waste products from the cells back to the heart.

> If the body's blood vessels were laid end to end, they'd cover about 60,000 miles — more than twice the circumference of the earth!

Between these two one-way street systems are tiny blood vessels called *capillaries*. Almost too tiny to see and often thinner than a strand of hair, capillaries connect the smallest arteries with the smallest veins. They are the bridges that connect our two systems of one-way streets. The walls of these tiny capillaries are so thin that food and oxygen in the blood pass through them into the surrounding cells. These thin walls also allow waste products from the cells to pass into the capillaries. This enables the blood to carry waste from the cells to be removed by the kidneys, liver, and lungs.

If you can imagine a single drop of blood flowing through this system, it might look something like this. The blood droplet, full of oxygen and nutrients (fuel), is pumped out of the left side of the heart into the largest arteries. There it flows into progressively smaller arteries and finally into the capillaries, where it delivers its load of oxygen and food for the cells. At the same time, the blood picks up waste products from the cells and flows into tiny veins, then into larger and larger veins. Finally, the blood droplet arrives back at the right side of the heart, where it's pumped into the lungs to unload carbon dioxide, pick up a fresh supply of oxygen, and begin its circular journey again.

The Heart: An Amazing Pump

The heart is the pump that keeps the blood flowing around and around in an endless circle throughout the body. Think of it as the traffic cop that coordinates the flow of traffic throughout our highway system. The heart is a hollow muscle that weighs less than a pound and is about the size of a man's fist. Despite its small size, this amazing organ beats an average of 100,000 times a day, pumping about two thousand gallons of blood every day. By the time you are seventy, your heart will have beaten more than 2.5 billion times.

Located in the center of the chest and protected by the breastbone and rib cage, the heart is actually a double pump that's divided into two upper chambers and two lower ones. A thin wall of tissue separates the left and right sides of the heart. The top chambers (*atriums* or *atria*) and lower chambers (*ventricles*) are connected by valves that act like one-way doors. These valves make sure blood flows only in one direction. In the heart, the blood is pumped from the left and right atriums to the left and right ventricles. The

Exterior of the Heart

Aorta

Arteries to Head and Arms

Pulmonary Artery

Superior Vena Cava

Left Atrium

Right Coronary Artery

Right Atrium

Left Anterior Descending Artery

Acute Marginal Artery

Left Ventricle

Inferior Vena Cava

Descending Aorta

Right Ventricle

right side of the heart sends blood to the lungs. The left side of the heart pumps blood out to the cells in the body.

Coronary Arteries

Just like other muscles in the body, the heart needs its own supply of blood and oxygen to work properly. Even though the heart pumps blood through its chambers, the heart itself receives no significant nourishment from this blood. A separate set of arteries that branch off the *aorta* (the main artery that receives blood from the left ventricle) provide the heart's blood supply. These are called *coronary arteries*. The coronary arteries encircle the top and sides of the heart, bringing it plenty of oxygen-rich blood. The two major coronary arteries are the *left coronary artery* and the *right coronary artery*. These vessels divide into many smaller coronary arteries that feed the heart.

> Arteries are strong and elastic, making them able to withstand pressure as the heart pumps. Veins have valves to help blood return to the heart.

What Causes Coronary Heart Disease?

Healthy coronary arteries have smooth, flexible walls that provide plenty of blood to the heart. However, over many years, these flexible walls can become progressively irritated and damaged by such substances as fats, cholesterol, calcium, cellular debris, and *platelets* (tiny cells responsible for blood clotting). When the walls of the arteries are damaged, these substances are able to "stick" to them. Coronary heart disease occurs when these coronary arteries become narrowed and clogged.

This buildup inside the artery walls is a process called ath-

Left: *Blocked artery.* Plaque buildup obstructs the flow of blood through this artery. The white area in the center is the only portion of the artery not blocked.

Right: *Normal artery.* The open artery, shown above, easily transports oxygenated blood away from the heart and to other parts of the body. *Photo courtesy of Custom Medical Stock Photo, Inc.*

erosclerosis, which produces a substance known as *plaque.* As it accumulates, plaque is a lot like the dirt, fat, and minerals that build up inside your home's plumbing. As the buildup becomes thicker, the flow through the pipes becomes less and less and may even completely stop. Similarly, when your heart doesn't get enough oxygen, due to narrowed arteries, you may feel chest pressure or pain called *angina.* If the blood supply to part of the heart is completely cut off, the result is often a *heart attack.*

Everyone has a certain amount of atherosclerosis as they age. For many of us, atherosclerosis begins in childhood. Some people have a rapid increase in the buildup of atherosclerotic plaque after age thirty. For others, plaque buildup doesn't become a problem until they're in their fifties or sixties.

You may hear the word *arteriosclerosis* being used interchangeably with atherosclerosis. The difference in the two words is technical. Arteriosclerosis refers to "hardening of the arteries." Atherosclerosis refers to the disease process by which plaque builds up in the arteries.

What Causes Atherosclerosis?

We don't know for sure why atherosclerosis occurs or even how it begins, but there are several theories. Some medical experts believe that the atherosclerotic buildup in the inner layers of the arteries may be caused by several conditions, including:

- elevated levels of LDL cholesterol (low-density lipoprotein) and triglycerides (a type of blood fat associated with CHD) in the blood
- low levels of HDL cholesterol (high-density lipoprotein)
- high blood pressure
- tobacco smoke
- high blood sugar levels (diabetes mellitus)
- inflammation

It's likely that more than one process is involved in the buildup of plaque. Many researchers believe that when excess fats combine with oxygen, they become trapped in the arterial wall. This attracts *white blood cells* which help prevent infection when tissue is damaged. Then substances called *prostaglandins*, which are involved in blood clotting and altering *tone* (firmness) within arteries, become active. Any injury to the artery wall, such as damage caused by smoking, can activate prostaglandins. The activated prostaglandins stimulate more plaque growth which narrows arteries and/or causes blood clots to form.

Regardless of how plaque forms, advanced plaque is made

up mostly of living cells. In fact, about 85 percent of advanced plaque consists of cell debris, calcium, smooth muscle cells, connective tissue, and *foam cells*, which are white blood cells that have digested fat. About 15 percent of advanced plaque is made up of fatty deposits.

Once the plaque develops, plaque containing cells can be easily damaged. This can lead to blood clots forming on the outside of the plaque. Small clots can further damage other layers of the blood vessel wall and stimulate more plaque growth. Larger blood clots can partially or totally block the artery.

In addition to interfering with or totally blocking blood flow, plaque can hinder the artery's ability to dilate and contract. In order to respond to the body's ever-changing need for blood, the arteries need to be strong and elastic. For instance, when you exercise, your body needs more blood. The heart responds by pumping faster, and the arteries respond by expanding to accommodate the increased volume of blood coming from the heart. As the artery becomes narrowed and hard, that elasticity is lost. Arteries that have atherosclerotic plaque are more apt to *spasm* (temporarily narrow), causing even less blood to flow to the heart and possibly causing chest pain or heart attack.

What is Metabolic Syndrome?

One of the conditions associated with the development of coronary heart disease is *metabolic syndrome*. Not an actual disease itself, metabolic syndrome is a cluster of disorders. According to current guidelines from the American Heart Association and National Cholesterol Education Program, you have metabolic syndrome if you have three or more of the following conditions:

- high fasting blood sugar levels
- high blood pressure
- low HDL cholesterol
- high triglycerides
- abdominal obesity—a waist circumference of forty inches or more in men, thirty-five inches or more in women.

Each of these disorders can lead to cardiovascular disease, stroke, and diabetes; however, the collective effect of metabolic syndrome significantly increases the risk of death from these diseases. One study reports that those with metabolic syndrome are 3.5 times more likely to die of a heart-related problem and five times as likely to develop type 2 diabetes.

The core disorder of metabolic syndrome is widely believed to be insulin resistance, which explains why the condition is sometimes referred to as *insulin resistance syndrome*. Insulin is a hormone that is supposed to help control the amount of sugar (*glucose*) in your bloodstream. When your body doesn't respond to the insulin the way it should, the result is higher levels of insulin and glucose in your blood. These higher levels lead to higher triglyceride levels and interfere with kidney function, which leads to increased blood pressure. The combination of these conditions leads to an increased risk for CHD.

How common is metabolic syndrome? Unfortunately, it's becoming increasingly common. It's estimated that 27 percent of the American population has metabolic syndrome. That's 55 million people. Two of the main factors that cause metabolic syndrome—obesity and physical inactivity—are related to lifestyle. Other factors include aging, genetic predisposition, hormonal imbalance, and a history of diabetes.

2 Risk Factors for Coronary Heart Disease

Y ou probably wonder why you developed coronary heart disease. We don't know exactly why some people develop CHD while others do not. We do know that certain traits or lifestyle habits—called *risk factors*—increase your chance of having a heart attack or stroke. The more risk factors you have, the higher the likelihood of you developing CHD. Many of the risk factors for heart attack and stroke also tend to speed up the rate at which atherosclerotic plaque builds up. That's why it's important to understand and control the risk factors for CHD. By controlling your risk factors you may be able to:

- slow down or even reverse the plaque building of atherosclerosis
- help prevent a heart attack or stroke

According to the National Heart, Lung, and Blood Institute of the National Institutes of Health, having multiple risk factors for CHD doesn't just add to your risk, it multiplies it. If, for instance, you're a smoker who has high blood pressure and high blood cholesterol, your risk for CHD is eight times greater than someone with no risk factors. *Major risk factors* are those that studies have shown significantly contribute to cardiovascular disease. Contributing risk factors are associated with increased risk, but more research needs to confirm their contribution to CHD. Most risk factors for CHD can be changed. Others, such as increasing age, family history, your race or gender, obviously, cannot.

Major CHD Risk Factors

Increasing Age

The older you are, the greater your risk for CHD, heart attack, and stroke. Four out of five people who die from CHD are sixty-five or older. If you're a man forty-five years or older, you're at increased risk for heart attack or stroke. If you're a woman fifty-five years or older, or you've passed menopause, or you've had your ovaries removed and you're not taking estrogen, you're at increased risk.

The aging process itself is partly to blame. As we age, the connective tissues in our artery walls naturally become less flexible. This is called *arteriosclerosis*, which as mentioned earlier, is "hardening of the arteries." This loss of flexibility in the arteries can cause blood pressure to increase, which can damage arteries and lead to the buildup of plaque. Rising blood pressure and hardened arteries can also make the heart work harder, which can cause the heart muscle to thicken and stiffen. Levels of blood cholesterol, another risk factor for CHD, also tend to rise with increasing age.

Family History of Heart Disease

If members of your family suffered from heart disease, you have a greater risk for CHD, heart attack, and stroke. You have even greater risk if your father or brother had a heart attack before age fifty-five or if your mother or sister had one before age sixty-five. You're also at increased risk if you have a relative who had a stroke.

Some people inherit genes that make them susceptible to the underlying causes of CHD such as diabetes, obesity, high blood cholesterol, or high blood pressure. For instance, diabetes or high blood pressure tends to run in some families. Other people may inherit risk factors such as *familial hypercholesterolemia*, a genetic disorder that causes excessively high LDL or "bad" blood cholesterol. For others, family lifestyle factors such as smoking, overeating, eating high-fat foods, and not exercising may contribute to increased risk.

Race

Some ethnic groups are at greater risk for CHD, heart attacks, and stroke. African Americans have

Major CHD Risk Factors

• Increasing age
• Family history of heart disease
• Race
• Male gender
• Personal history of heart disease
• High blood cholesterol
• Smoking
• High blood pressure
• Being overweight
• Physical inactivity
• Diabetes

Contributing CHD Risk Factors

• Stress
• Hormonal factors
• Birth control pills
• Excessive alcohol use
• Elevated homocysteine levels

higher rates of high blood pressure, a major risk factor for CHD. Mexican Americans, Native Americans, native Hawaiians, and some Asian Americans also have a higher risk for heart disease. Heart experts suspect higher risk among people in these groups may be related, in part, to their increased rates of obesity, diabetes, and cigarette smoking. Economic disadvantages and lack of access to good health care may also play a part in higher rates of heart disease and poorer prognosis among some groups. In Japan, the incidence of CHD is lower than in Western countries, yet when Japanese immigrate to North America, their CHD risk climbs, though not as high as other Americans. This suggests that both genetics (race) and environment play a role in CHD.

Male Gender

Men have a greater chance of having a heart attack and having one earlier than women. Although this may be due to hormonal differences between men and women, men's rates of heart disease are greater even when compared to postmenopausal women who have lost their gender protection against heart attack.

Personal History of Heart Disease

If you have CHD, you're at increased risk for a heart attack or stroke. If you've already had a heart attack, you're at increased risk for having a second one.

High Blood Cholesterol

Cholesterol is a waxy, fatlike substance that's found in every cell in the body. It's a necessary substance that helps digest fats, strengthens cell membranes (linings), and makes up part of some types of hormones and vitamins (e.g., vitamin D). However, too much cholesterol (*hyperlipidemia*) can be bad for you, causing artery-clogging plaque.

Having high blood cholesterol is one of the most important risk factors for CHD and subsequent heart attacks and strokes. However, risk depends on the *type* of cholesterol you have. The higher your level of *LDL cholesterol* (low-density lipoprotein)—"bad" cholesterol—the greater your risk. When you have too much LDL cholesterol in your blood, the excess builds up on the walls of the coronary arteries. The opposite is true for "good" cholesterol, *HDL cholesterol* (high-density lipoprotein): having high HDL cholesterol protects against CHD; having low HDL cholesterol is a CHD risk factor.

You get cholesterol in two ways: from the liver and from foods you eat. The liver produces all the cholesterol your body needs. Many of the foods we eat, such as egg yolks, meats, poultry, and whole dairy products, contain cholesterol. Eating too many of these foods can cause high blood cholesterol. As mentioned earlier in this chapter, you can also develop high blood cholesterol if you have certain genetic factors such as familial hypercholesterolemia. Because high blood cholesterol is such a major risk factor, we'll talk more about it in chapter 3.

Smoking

The American Heart Association calls smoking "the single most preventable cause of death in the United States." Thirty percent of all deaths from CHD in the United States are caused by smoking. In fact, smokers' risk of heart attack is double that of nonsmokers. Smokers who have heart attacks are twice as likely to die and die suddenly (within an hour) than nonsmokers. If you smoke and have other CHD risk factors, you significantly multiply your risk. For those with advanced atherosclerosis, smoking is especially dangerous.

According to a number of studies, including the famous Framingham Heart Study, smoking is a powerful risk factor for CHD and heart attack. When you smoke or are exposed to secondhand smoke:

- blood pressure, heart rate, and the amount of blood pumped by the heart temporarily rise, which causes the heart to work harder.
- arteries in the legs and arms constrict (narrow).
- delicate tissues inside the arteries become damaged and are more subject to the buildup of artery-clogging plaque.
- blood supply to the heart, especially in the tiny vessels supplying the heart muscle, decreases.
- platelets, the clotting agents in blood, become stickier and tend to clump together, so the blood becomes thicker and clotting time is reduced.
- plaques that are already built up in the arteries can become destabilized. This promotes *rupture* (cracks in the inner walls of a blood vessel) and the formation of blood clots (*thrombi*) inside a blood vessel or chamber of the heart.
- "bad" LDL cholesterol levels increase, and "good" HDL cholesterol levels in the blood decrease.

Blood Pressure Guidelines

Classification	Systolic Pressure	Diastolic Pressure
Normal	less than 120	less than 80
High Normal (Prehypertension)	120–139	80–89
High Blood Pressure		
Stage 1	140–159	90–99
Stage 2	160–179	100–109
Stage 3	180 or higher	110 or higher

High Blood Pressure (HBP)

Blood pressure is the measurement of the force when the heart pumps blood into the arteries and out to the body *and* the force placed on the arteries as they resist the blood from the heart. It is written as two numbers—*systolic* (top number) and *diastolic* (bottom number)—expressed in millimeters of mercury (mmHg). The National Institutes of Health Joint National Committee on Blood Pressure has created categories for blood pressure. The higher your blood pressure, the greater your risk for CHD, heart attack, and other health problems.

When your blood pressure is too high (140/90 mmHg or higher), also called *hypertension*, your heart has to work harder. Over time, this can cause the heart muscle to become larger and thicker and may ultimately weaken the heart, making it unable to meet the body's need for blood and oxygen (*heart failure*).

High blood pressure (HBP) damages the arteries and arterioles, scarring them and making them hard and less elastic. It also speeds up the buildup of atherosclerotic plaque and may lead to heart attacks. As arteries become narrower, clots are more likely to form and block the blood supply completely.

If you have HBP and other CHD risk factors such as obesity, smoking, diabetes, and/or high blood cholesterol, your risk multiplies. HBP is also associated with stroke, kidney failure, and serious eye damage.

Being Overweight

Being overweight increases your risk for CHD and heart attack as well as for a number of other health problems. If you carry your excess weight around your waist (the so-called apple shape), your heart disease risk is even higher. Being overweight:

- forces the heart to work harder
- raises blood pressure
- increases blood cholesterol and trigylcerides (a type of blood fat)
- lowers "good" HDL blood cholesterol
- increases the risk for developing diabetes, another risk factor for CHD

Physical Inactivity

If you're a couch potato, you're at risk for heart disease and heart attack. Heart experts have determined that being inactive is a major risk for heart disease/heart attack. The risk may be as high as six times that of those who are active.

If you don't exercise and you overeat, you may be putting yourself at even greater risk. Not exercising and overeating may cause you to become overweight, have high blood pressure and/or high blood cholesterol, and develop diabetes—all important risk factors for CHD and heart attack.

Diabetes

Diabetes mellitus is a problem with the body's metabolism, or energy-burning system. When you have diabetes, your body isn't able to produce and/or properly respond to the hormone *insulin*. Insulin allows your body to convert blood sugar (*glucose*) into energy. Diabetes is also a major risk factor for heart disease and heart attacks. Two-thirds of people with diabetes die from some form of heart or blood vessel disease.

Type 2 diabetes, or *adult-onset diabetes*, is the type that often develops around middle age. Being overweight and inactive are two risk factors that put you at risk for developing diabetes. Many people who have mild type 2 diabetes don't even know it for many years. Untreated, diabetes can cause a number of serious health problems, including blood vessel disease that can affect the eyes and kidneys.

Even when your diabetes is treated and you have your blood glucose levels under control, having diabetes significantly increases your risk for heart disease and stroke. One of the reasons for this may be that diabetes affects blood cholesterol and *triglyceride* levels (triglycerides are a type of blood fat associated with CHD). In addition, people with diabetes often have high blood pressure, another major risk factor for CHD and heart attacks.

Contributing CHD Risk Factors

The following risk factors are associated with CHD and heart attack, but additional research needs to be done to find out exactly *how*, and *how much*, they contribute to the CHD/heart attack equation.

Stress

All of us have stress in our lives and everyone reacts to stress a little differently. Some people are cool and calm most of the time. Stressful events don't seem to faze them much. Others have a "shorter fuse" and tend to overreact to the smallest stresses. While heart experts aren't all in agreement about the correlation between heart disease and how we react to stress, a growing body of evidence suggests that those who react more negatively to stress (for example, becoming angry or depressed) may be at greater risk for heart problems. A six-year study conducted at the University of North Carolina at Chapel Hill found those who were prone to anger were three times more likely to have a heart attack or sudden cardiac death than those who weren't anger-prone. At a recent annual meeting of the American College of Cardiology, researchers from Johns Hopkins reported similar results. They found that people who reacted to stress in a hot-tempered manner were nineteen times more likely to suffer *ischemia* (reduced blood flow to the heart), and their coronary arteries and other blood vessels stayed constricted for an abnormally long period of time.

We don't know if stress is an independent risk factor for CHD or if it simply affects other CHD risk factors such as high blood pressure. We do know that stress may cause a person to adopt unhealthful behaviors such as overeating or cigarette smoking, both of which can contribute to heart disease.

Hormonal Factors

Sex hormones affect one's risk for CHD and heart attacks. It's well known that men suffer more heart attacks and suffer them about ten years earlier than women. Female hormones tend to raise "good" HDL cholesterol and reduce "bad" LDL cholesterol. In contrast, male hormones do just the opposite.

A number of studies suggest that after menopause the loss of natural estrogen puts women at higher risk for CHD and heart attack. Women who undergo surgical menopause by the removal of the uterus and ovaries and who do not take replacement hormones have a dramatic rise in heart attack risk (similar to men's risk).

Birth Control Pills

Early forms of birth control pills often contained high doses of estrogen. While women's natural female hormones have a heart-protective effect, inexplicably, high estrogen-dose birth control pills do not. These birth control pills are associated with an increased risk for heart attack and stroke, especially among older women who smoke cigarettes. Newer forms of birth control pills contain less estrogen and therefore have a much lower risk.

Women who smoke and take birth control pills—even newer, lower-dose ones—are at higher risk for developing blood clots. After age thirty-five, smoking and taking birth control pills increases heart attack risk even more.

Excessive Alcohol Use

We have all heard that drinking a small amount of alcohol may lower the risk of heart disease. However, drinking excessively (more than one drink per day for women, more than two drinks per day for men) increases heart disease risk. Drinking too much alcohol can increase blood pressure, a major risk factor for CHD and heart attack. Excessive drinking has been associated with irregular heartbeats and high triglycerides, a type of blood fat that may contribute to CHD. Excessive drinking can cause heart failure, a condition in which the heart is unable to pump enough blood to supply all the parts of the body. Alcohol also contributes to obesity, another major CHD risk factor.

Elevated Homocysteine Levels

Homocysteine is an *amino acid,* or protein building block. It is a natural by-product of the body's breakdown of protein. We know that homocysteine is necessary for the production of two other amino acids, *cysteine* and *methionine.* Low intakes of folate, vitamin B_6, and vitamin B_{12} are associated with higher levels of homocysteine.

For more than thirty years, researchers have speculated that elevated levels of homocysteine may be a cause of atherosclerosis. Research in the past ten years confirms that elevated levels of homocysteine is associated with CHD. Thirty percent of the heart patients in the Framingham Heart Study had elevated levels of homocysteine.

It's not known precisely how elevated levels of homocysteine relate to heart disease. One theory suggests that high levels causes blood vessel walls to narrow. Homocysteine may also encourage the development of blood clots by interfering with a natural anticoagulant, *protein C.*

3 The Cholesterol–Coronary Heart Disease Connection

Numerous research studies have established that abnormalities in cholesterol, particularly high LDL cholesterol and low HDL cholesterol, play a major role in the development of CHD and heart attacks. Cholesterol is one of the major components of artery-clogging plaque, so it's important to understand cholesterol's relationship to heart disease.

As mentioned in chapter 2, the waxy, fatlike substance cholesterol is necessary for life. However, the body needs only a small amount of cholesterol. The liver produces about 1,000 milligrams of cholesterol every day, or about 80 percent of your blood cholesterol. That's all the cholesterol your body really needs.

However, we also get cholesterol from foods that come from animals, such as meats, poultry, fish, egg yolks, and whole milk products. About 20 percent of our blood cholesterol comes from dietary cholesterol. The amount of fat and cholesterol you eat can influence all your blood fats, including blood cholesterol levels.

The problem occurs when there's too much cholesterol circulating in the bloodstream. As you now know, excess cholesterol can lead to atherosclerosis, the plaque-building process that narrows arteries throughout the body and can lead to chest pain, heart attack, or stroke.

Types of Cholesterol

Everyone knows that oil and water do not mix. The same is true for cholesterol and blood. Cholesterol cannot dissolve in blood. To enable cholesterol to travel through the blood, the body coats cholesterol with proteins called *apoproteins*. Once combined with the protein, a complex called a *lipoprotein* is formed. These protein carriers transport cholesterol and triglycerides (another type of blood fat) through the bloodstream. There are several different types of lipoproteins. Each affects CHD and heart attack risk differently.

> More than half of all Americans have total cholesterol levels higher than 200 mg/dL, putting them at increased risk for CHD and heart attack.

Low-Density Lipoprotein (LDL) Cholesterol

This type of lipoprotein is called "bad" cholesterol because it is the main source of cholesterol in the blood and one of the major culprits in the buildup of atherosclerotic plaque. (Remember that LDL is the "bad" cholesterol by associating the L with "lousy.") LDL cholesterol carries some 60 to 70 percent of the body's circulating cholesterol.

As LDL cholesterol circulates through the bloodstream, the body uses some of it to build cells. Some of the cholesterol returns to the liver. However, when there is too much LDL cholesterol circulating in the blood, it can slowly build up on the walls of the coronary arteries. The more LDL cholesterol you have in your blood, the higher your risk for CHD and heart attack.

High-Density Lipoprotein (HDL) Cholesterol

This is the so-called "good" cholesterol (remember that HDL is the "good" cholesterol by associating the H with "healthy"). High-density lipoprotein particles, which contain mostly protein, carry anywhere from 20 to 30 percent of the cholesterol in the blood. HDL cholesterol is considered "good" because it acts like a trash collector, picking up excess cholesterol from the artery walls and sending it to the liver for disposal. Thus, HDL cholesterol slows plaque growth and may reverse the plaque-building process. The higher your level of HDL, the lower your risk of heart disease and heart attack. Conversely, low levels of HDL increase your risk for CHD and heart attack.

Very Low-Density Lipoprotein (VLDL) Cholesterol

The largest of the lipoproteins, VLDL contains about 15 percent of the blood's cholesterol and most of the triglycerides. A significant amount of VLDL is converted to LDL cholesterol. Consequently, some types of VLDL cholesterol may contribute to plaque building.

Triglycerides

Triglycerides are another type of blood fat. Most of the body's fat is stored as triglycerides in fat tissue. A small portion of triglycerides circulate in the blood. Triglyceride levels in the blood are related to how much and what kind of dietary fat and carbohydrates (sugar and starches) and how much alcohol you consume. Triglyceride levels are also influenced by genetics.

Heart experts believe that excessive levels of triglycerides may contribute to the fatty deposits that obstruct blood flow and increase the risk for heart attack. A twenty-year study recently published in the journal *Circulation* found that people with elevated triglycerides have a greater risk of dying from a heart attack, even if their blood cholesterol is normal.

The Problem of Unstable Plaques

As excess cholesterol travels in the blood, it is taken up by special cells in the artery walls. This process creates "lumps" in the artery walls that are covered over or encapsulated by fibrous scar tissue. Some of these so-called *stable plaques* become quite large and dramatically narrow or even totally block arteries. When these large blockages reduce the amount of blood getting to the heart, they can cause chest pain, or angina.

However, it is the smaller, *unstable plaques*, which are thinly or not entirely covered over by scar tissue, that pose the biggest threat for heart attacks. These plaques are loaded with cholesterol and have a tendency to rupture easily. When these unstable plaques burst into the artery channel (*lumen*), they release their cholesterol back into the local bloodstream. The body responds by triggering a blood clot inside the artery to repair the perceived damage to the inner artery wall. This blood clot may totally block the artery, stopping blood flow and causing a heart attack. The area of the heart that doesn't receive blood starts to die within twenty minutes, permanently damaging the heart muscle. Even if the clot doesn't cause a heart attack, it can cause electrical disturbances that interfere with the heart's rhythm (*arrhythmias*). This condition can lead to cardiac arrest (sudden stopping of the heart) and death.

Reducing the amount of cholesterol in the blood can help lower the amount of cholesterol in plaques, making them more stable and less likely to burst and trigger a heart attack. Even in people who have already had a heart attack, lowering cholesterol can lower the chance of having another heart attack in the future.

What Constitutes High Cholesterol?

Doctors measure blood levels of total cholesterol, HDL and LDL cholesterol, and triglycerides to assess the risk of atherosclerosis and heart attack. Previously, heart experts recommended that people without heart disease have their total cholesterol and HDL cholesterol tested every five years. However, we now recognize that because LDL is a major cause of CHD, it is also important to measure LDL.

According to guidelines from the National Heart, Lung, and Blood Institute's National Cholesterol Education Program Expert Panel (NCEP), all adults over age twenty should have their total cholesterol, HDL and LDL cholesterol, and triglyceride levels checked at least once every five years. Doctors call this test a *lipoprotein* or *lipid profile*.

Factors Contributing to High Cholesterol

In most cases, there is no single cause of high blood cholesterol. Your blood cholesterol level may certainly be affected by your diet. But it may also be affected by how quickly your body makes LDL cholesterol and how rapidly it gets rid of it.

Genetics

Genes you inherit from your family can influence how rapidly your body makes LDL cholesterol and how efficiently it's removed. Your liver might produce too many VLDL particles or too few HDL particles, making you prone to high cholesterol. Some people—

Classification of HDL Cholesterol Levels	
High	60 mg/dL (desired level; higher is better)
Low	less than 40 mg/dL

Classification of LDL Cholesterol Levels	
Ideal	less than 70 mg/dL
Normal	70–100 mg/dL
Borderline High	101–130 mg/dL
High	131–160 mg/dL
Very High	greater than 160 mg/dL

Note: Measurements are expressed in milligrams per deciliter of blood.

approximately one in 500—have familial hypercholesterolemia, an inherited disorder that causes cholesterol levels to be extremely high (350 to 500 mg/dL). Even if you don't have an inherited cholesterol disorder, your genetics influence your cholesterol levels.

Diet

What you eat influences your blood cholesterol levels, too. How much saturated fat (a type of fat that comes mostly in foods from animals, such as meat, egg yolks, and dairy products) and dietary cholesterol you eat can raise or lower your cholesterol levels.

Calorie Balance and Your Weight

Calorie balance refers to the number of calories you take in versus the number of calories you burn each day. When you take in more calories than you burn, you gain weight. Excess weight tends to increase LDL cholesterol levels. When your extra pounds are around your waist, your risk for heart disease is even greater. Losing weight can lower "bad" LDL cholesterol levels, raise "good" HDL cholesterol, and reduce triglyceride levels.

Physical Activity

Inactivity can negatively influence your blood cholesterol levels. Regular physical activity can decrease "bad" VLDL cholesterol, raise "good" HDL cholesterol levels, and, in some people, even lower "bad" LDL cholesterol levels.

Age

As people get older, their blood cholesterol levels tend to rise. This rise usually levels off at about sixty to sixty-five years of age.

Factors Affecting Cholesterol

- Genetics
- Diet
- Calorie balance and your weight
- Physical activity
- Age
- Menopause
- Smoking
- Diabetes
- Stress

Menopause

Women's total blood cholesterol levels tend to be lower than those for men of the same age. However, after menopause, women's LDL cholesterol increases and their HDL cholesterol tends to decrease. Some authorities believe this change in cholesterol levels may be why women's risk of heart disease rises sharply after menopause.

Smoking

In addition to damaging blood vessel walls and making them more susceptible to the development of atherosclerotic plaque, smoking can lower "good" HDL cholesterol levels by as much as 15 percent.

Diabetes

In many people, diabetes can increase triglycerides and decrease "good" HDL cholesterol levels.

Stress

While it's hard to pin down the impact of stress in heart disease, some studies indicate that over a long period of time stress raises blood cholesterol levels. It's unclear whether this rise is due to the direct effect stress has on the body's chemistry, or whether it's because stress may influence people to indulge in behaviors such as smoking and overeating that are risky for the heart.

4   Symptoms of Coronary Heart Disease

Symptoms are subjective changes in the way the body feels that may signal illness or disease. A symptom isn't a disease itself, but a feeling or complaint indicating something is wrong. You may have coronary heart disease and not even know it. Especially in the early stages of CHD, you may have no symptoms at all. You may feel fine, unaware that there's a silent time bomb ticking away inside your coronary arteries. As the arteries become narrower and the heart begins to have less and less blood and oxygen available to it, you may experience shortness of breath or angina—periodic pain, tightness, or pressure in the chest. Some people may develop no symptoms. Their first indication that they have CHD is a potentially deadly heart attack.

Chest Pain and/or Angina Pectoris

Pressure, pain, and/or tightness in the chest is the symptom most commonly associated with CHD. Known as *angina* or *angina pectoris*, this pain occurs when the heart doesn't receive enough blood and oxygen. It is often a recurring pain or discomfort in the chest that occurs when part of the heart doesn't get enough blood. People often describe angina as pressure, squeezing, burning, tightness, or heaviness. Most commonly the discomfort is felt under the breastbone. However, sometimes people feel discomfort in the shoulders, arms, neck, jaw, or back. Some people also experience numbness in the shoulders, arms, or wrists.

Angina usually lasts no more than five to fifteen minutes. Events that may trigger angina include: exertion or physical stress (times when the heart's demand for oxygen increases), eating a heavy meal, exposure to extreme heat or cold, drinking alcohol, and cigarette smoking. Angina may be relieved within a few minutes by stopping the stressful activity.

Angina is *not* a heart attack. During an episode of angina, a reduction in blood flow to the heart causes discomfort. Angina attacks usually do not permanently damage the heart muscle. In contrast, during a heart attack, blood flow to part of the heart is partially or completely blocked. The pain during a heart attack is usually more severe and lasts longer, and the damage to the heart muscle may be serious and is permanent.

But chest pain may also be caused by other serious heart and circulatory problems: pericarditis, dissection of the aorta, or pulmonary embolism.

Pericarditis is an inflammation of the *pericardium*, the fibrous outer sac that surrounds the heart. The chest pain it causes is usually sharp, even knifelike. It's made worse by taking a deep breath or lying down and gets better when you lean forward.

Dissection of the aorta is a tearing of the inner lining of the major artery that leads away from the heart. The pain, often described as a tearing sensation, can be excruciating.

A *pulmonary embolism* is a blood clot in the lung. The pain is located in the chest and typically gets worse when you take a deep breath, or it may cause chest heaviness that's identical to angina. Both angina and pulmonary emboli may cause some degree of breathlessness.

Non-heart problems may also cause pain and discomfort similar to angina. For instance, gallbladder disease or inflammation of the esophagus from the reflux of stomach acid, often referred to as GERD (gastroesophageal reflux disease), both cause chest pain. Problems in the joints, nerves, or chest wall can also cause angina-like pain.

Types of Angina

We classify angina as stable or unstable. If you have *stable angina*, you probably experience chest discomfort when you overexert. The pain is relatively predictable and, almost any time you overexert, the pain comes back. For instance, you may feel chest pain and tightness when you perform heavy labor such as shoveling snow or during times of emotional stress. Over time, you probably learn to identify what brings on your angina attacks.

Unstable angina is less predictable. It includes:

- new chest pain or discomfort that may come on suddenly during activities that never caused problems before
- a changing pattern of stable angina (pain occurring at lower levels of activity, more often, or more severely)
- chest pain that occurs at rest or that wakes one from sleep

Unstable angina is more dangerous because it carries a higher risk of heart attack. Although both stable and unstable anginas are caused by the atherosclerotic plaques of CHD, the plaque in unstable angina is more often related to rupturing on the inner surface of the artery. When this happens, the body forms a blood clot to repair the damage. If the clot is large enough, it may block blood flow and cause a heart attack. Unstable angina can also cause severe heart rhythm problems or sudden cardiac death, in which the heart muscle simply stops functioning.

> Take angina seriously, especially if you smoke, are overweight, have a family history of heart disease, have high cholesterol, are diabetic, or have high blood pressure.

A third, less common type of angina is called *variant* or *Prinzmetal's angina*. In this form of angina, the muscle fibers surrounding the coronary arteries go into spasm, which causes a blood vessel to become very narrow or even close off completely. About 65 percent of people who suffer variant angina have severe coronary atherosclerotic plaque in at least one major coronary vessel. The spasm usually occurs very close to the artery blockage. Variant angina attacks often occur without exertion or other apparent cause, or they may be brought on by stress, exposure to cold, or cigarette smoking. Variant angina attacks are usually severe and last only a short time. They often occur between midnight and 8:00 A.M., waking the person from sleep with the discomfort. During attacks, abnormal heart rhythms can cause the person to lose consciousness.

The Heart's Warning

Regardless of the type of angina you may have, it has the same cause: not enough oxygen getting to the heart due to atherosclerotic plaque. Angina is a warning from your heart. Angina may not indicate that you are about to have a heart attack, but it does mean that you have underlying CHD and that you may be at increased risk for heart attack. If you experience angina:

Don't ignore it. Angina is your body's cry for help. See your doctor *immediately* for evaluation. Don't wait a few days or a few weeks for an appointment to address the symptoms. Once your condition is properly diagnosed, your doctor can prescribe lifestyle changes, medication, or medical procedures such as angioplasty to relieve your discomfort.

Know what angina is. Not all chest pain is angina. The pain is probably *not* angina if:

- it lasts for less than 30 seconds
- taking a deep breath relieves it
- it goes away after drinking a glass of water
- it disappears if you change body positions
- it's localized on the surface of your chest and you can reproduce it by touching a particular spot

If you have any doubt, see your doctor. Remember, it's better to have the problem checked out early.

Learn the pattern of your angina. Once your doctor has evaluated and treated your condition, try to learn what brings on and what relieves attacks. Pay attention to what your angina attacks feel like, how long episodes usually last, and how medication affects them.

Watch for changes. When the pattern of angina changes, the risk of heart attack increases for days or even weeks. See your doctor right away if your angina:

- becomes more frequent
- lasts longer
- occurs at rest

Know the symptoms of a heart attack. See the list of symptoms later in this chapter and commit it to memory. Call for emergency medical help (911 in most areas) immediately if the pattern of your angina changes sharply or if you have any symptoms of heart attack.

Treatment for Angina

In chapter 7, we cover medications used to treat angina; however, there is also a nonmedication treatment for the condition. It can be used as an alternative to medication or in conjunction with it. The procedure, called *enhanced external counterpulsation (EECP)*, is used to provide relief for symptoms of angina. The treatments, usually administered as a series, aim for long-lasting improvement in blood flow, which increases exercise tolerance. Some people have experienced positive effects for up to five years following treatment.

The treatment, which isn't painful but can be uncomfortable, involves placing long inflatable cuffs (similar to blood pressure cuffs) around each of your legs while you're lying down. As each heartbeat begins, the cuffs deflate, and as each heartbeat ends, they inflate. This "milking" action increases blood flow into the coronary arteries while reducing the amount of work required by your heart. These actions reduce cardiac ischemia.

Although EECP can be beneficial for most people, it isn't for everyone. You may not be suitable for EECP if you have any of the following conditions:

- recent catheterization
- arrhythmia
- severe high blood pressure
- valvular heart disease
- history of blood clots in the legs
- blockages in the leg arteries

Even though studies have shown that the therapy can be effective, it's still scientifically unclear why the benefits of EECP continue after the treatment is finished. Because of this, many doctors remain skeptical of it. As a result, the treatment is recommended selectively, and cardiologists offer it in their offices.

Silent Ischemia

When there is a temporary shortage of blood and oxygen to the heart without any symptoms, it's called *silent ischemia*. It can occur when a coronary artery is narrowed by atherosclerotic plaque, or spasm, or a combination of the two. The problem with silent ischemia is that there's no pain, no discomfort, no warning—until there's a heart attack. It's like a smoke detector that's been disconnected—it prevents the alarm being sounded when a fire breaks out.

Heart Attack

Doctors call a heart attack a *coronary attack* or *myocardial infarction (MI)*. Other names for it include *coronary occlusion* or *coronary thrombosis*. Basically, these all mean the same thing.

A heart attack occurs when the blood supply to part of the heart is severely reduced or completely blocked. This occurs when one of the coronary arteries supplying the heart becomes severely narrowed or blocked, usually from a combination of too much atherosclerotic plaque and a blood clot. Typically, when plaque tears or ruptures, the cholesterol core of the plaque is exposed to circulating blood cells (platelets). In response, the body forms a blood clot. If this blood clot severely restricts or blocks the blood supply to part of the heart, a heart attack can occur.

Sixty percent of people who die of a heart attack die within the first hour. Get help fast! Time is critical in a heart attack.

If heart cells are denied blood and oxygen for a prolonged period of time, they suffer irreversible injury and begin to die. Depending on how much of the heart is damaged, a heart attack can cause the heart to be unable to pump enough blood to the body (heart failure) or cause death.

Heart attacks can also occur when a coronary artery temporarily goes into spasm. This can reduce or even stop blood flow to part of the heart, especially if the coronary artery is already narrowed by atherosclerotic plaque. Many factors contribute to spasm, including the local release of chemical substances that may trigger spasm and the sensitivity of the artery to contract. Both normal and diseased arteries may develop spasm. If the spasm is severe enough, a heart attack can result.

Common Heart Attack Symptoms

- uncomfortable pressure, tightness, fullness, squeezing, or pain in the center of the chest
- pain that lasts more than a few minutes (thirty minutes to

several hours) or goes away and comes back
- pain that spreads to the shoulders, neck, or arms
- light-headedness or fainting
- nausea
- profuse sweating
- shortness of breath

Less Typical Signs of a Heart Attack

Not everyone experiences a heart attack the same way. Even if you've had one or more heart attacks, another attack may feel different. Some people feel the classic, heavy, heart attack chest pain. People often describe it as a "vice squeezing my chest." Others may have only a vague sense of discomfort, indigestion, breathlessness, and/or dizziness. People who have diabetes, women, and people over the age of seventy-five often have symptoms that are less typical, such as:

- vague chest pain
- stomach or abdominal pain
- nausea or dizziness, without chest pain
- shortness of breath or difficulty breathing, without chest pain
- anxiety without obvious cause, impending sense of doom
- weakness or fatigue
- erratic heartbeat
- cold sweating
- paleness
- frequent angina not caused by exertion
- dry mouth or cough, usually with breathlessness

Immediate Medical Care Is Critical

With heart attacks, time is critical. The longer the artery is blocked, the more damage to the heart muscle and the greater the risk of permanent disability or even death. Additionally, a heart attack can cause the electrical signals of the heart that regulate its rhythm and pumping to become scrambled. Instead of pumping in a synchronized fashion, the heart twitches erratically (*ventricular fibrillation*) and becomes unable to pump blood. If ventricular fibrillation lasts longer than a few minutes, it can cause death. Many people mistake the symptoms of a heart attack for indigestion or stress and they delay getting to the hospital. This is a dangerous and often fatal mistake. *Anyone who experiences heart attack symptoms should be rushed to the nearest hospital* (they should *not* drive themselves).

Remember this important tip. Chewing aspirin during a heart attack can save your life.

If you get to an emergency room fast, doctors can use a variety of techniques and medications to help restore blood flow to the part of the heart that is damaged during the heart attack. Called *reperfusion therapy*, this may involve clot-dissolving medications, balloon angioplasty (and stenting), or surgery. Restoring the heart's blood flow is vitally important because damage to even less than 10 percent of the ventricle muscle decreases the amount of blood your heart can pump with each beat. If 25 percent or more of the heart muscle is damaged, your heart can enlarge and be unable to pump adequately (heart failure). When 40 percent or more of the heart muscle is damaged, shock or death may result. The sooner the doctors can use reperfusion techniques on your heart, the more likely you'll survive. In fact, one study by the University of Washington showed that three-quarters of people survived heart attacks with little or no heart damage when they received clot-dissolving therapy within seventy minutes of the beginning of symptoms. New and better blood thinners are continuing to improve these results.

The results are even better when there's an experienced cardiologist available at the hospital to perform direct angioplasty (a procedure that opens the arteries) and stenting (propping open the arteries with fine wire mesh). Ideally, this procedure should be completed within ninety minutes after arriving at an emergency room. This approach can reduce death rates from heart attacks to less than 5 percent at a six-month follow-up. We'll talk more about these two procedures in chapter 8.

Surviving a Heart Attack

Knowing what to do in the case of a heart attack can mean the difference in life and death. The following guidelines can help save the life of someone having a heart attack.

- Keep a list of emergency rescue numbers handy. Call 911 or other emergency medical number immediately if you experience symptoms.
- Know which medical centers offer twenty-four-hour cardiac care and which one is closest to your home and office.
- Know and recognize the symptoms of heart attack. About half of all heart attack victims have warning signs hours, days, or even weeks before an attack. Be aware that not all heart attacks involve the classic crushing chest pain.
- Chew one regular-strength aspirin if you experience heart attack symptoms. It will help break up clots if you're having an attack. When taken during an attack, aspirin can decrease death rates by about 25 percent. Chewing the

aspirin speeds its absorption. If you're not having a heart attack, it likely will not hurt you.

- If your doctor has given you nitroglycerine tablets, place one under your tongue when symptoms begin. Repeat every five minutes for a total of three doses. (Do *not* take nitroglycerine if your doctor hasn't prescribed it for you or if you feel dizzy, unless you're directly supervised by a health-care professional. Taking nitroglycerine for some types of heart conditions can be dangerous. Do *not* take nitroglycerine if you have taken *Viagra*, *Cialis*, or *Levitra* within twenty-four hours.

- If you can't get ambulance service, have someone drive you (don't drive yourself) to the nearest emergency medical facility.

- Have someone close to you trained in *cardiopulmonary resuscitation (CPR)*. You may need it if your heart stops beating. CPR can help parts of your body receive oxygen until emergency medical help arrives.

Sudden Cardiac Death

Sudden cardiac death (SCD) is the most common reason people die from CHD. SCD is the abrupt, total loss of heart function (*cardiac arrest*) in someone with or without diagnosed heart disease. Death is unexpected. About half of all deaths from atherosclerosis are from SCD.

People who die from SCD almost always have underlying heart disease. Most often, it is atherosclerosis. In about 90 percent of those who die from SCD, two or more major coronary arteries are narrowed by atherosclerotic plaque. Two-thirds of SCD victims have heart damage from previous heart attacks. The first six months following a heart attack is a high-risk time for people to die from SCD.

SCD has the same risk factors as CHD. Strategies to reduce risk factors for CHD and reduce/prevent atherosclerosis can help reduce the risk of dying from SCD.

5 Women and Coronary Heart Disease

Many women believe that coronary heart disease is "a man's problem." Nothing could be further from the truth. Heart disease (especially CHD) and stroke are the leading causes of death for women in the United States and in most developed countries. Every year, heart disease and stroke kills more than half a million women in the United States, nearly twice as many as from all forms of cancer, including breast cancer. In fact, twice as many women die from heart disease as from breast cancer. The risk is even greater for minority women. The rate of death from heart disease for black women is 69 percent higher than for white women. Black women are more likely to die of a heart attack before menopause, too.

Unfortunately, most women are not aware of their risk for heart disease. A recent poll conducted for the American Heart Association found that most women do not recognize that heart disease is women's leading health problem and their number one cause of death today. In fact, fewer than one in ten women believe heart disease is their greatest health threat.

Although CHD is the number one cause of death for women,

a woman's first clue might be a full-blown, potentially fatal heart attack (or stroke if the blockage occurs in the brain). That's because the artery-clogging plaque building of atherosclerosis is invisible. Over a lifetime, plaque deposits build silently. Two-thirds of women who die of a heart attack have no prior symptoms, compared to only half of men.

CHD isn't just a disease of older women. Certainly, women over sixty-five are most vulnerable to CHD. However, middle-aged women between forty-five and sixty-four are at risk, too. One in nine American women in this age group show signs of CHD.

Diagnosis Differences in Women and Men

While women don't recognize the threat CHD poses, health experts have also been slow to recognize and respond to the problem of heart disease in women. Many of the studies on heart disease have been conducted on male subjects. Only in the last few years have studies taken place that will clarify how heart disease manifests itself differently in the sexes. The results of this research will improve diagnostic and treatment strategies for women.

In a survey of nearly 30,000 office visits, the Centers for Disease Control and Prevention found that doctors are less likely to provide women than men with information about heart-healthy nutrition, exercise, and weight reduction. This is disturbing news considering that:

- Obesity is increasing.
- Approximately 25 percent of women report they get no regular physical activity.
- Approximately 52 percent of women older than forty-five have elevated blood pressure.

- Nearly 40 percent of women fifty-five and older have elevated blood cholesterol levels.
- Smoking rates for women are declining less than for men.

Women are also less likely than men to get the right diagnosis and treatment for CHD. The American Heart Association concluded that both women and their doctors often attribute chest pains to non-heart causes, resulting in dangerous misdiagnoses. Part of this may be due to the fact that women are more apt to have subtle, atypical heart attack symptoms. While some women have the classic heart attack chest pain that radiates to the shoulders, neck, or arms, many have less typical chest discomfort or abdominal pain, difficulty breathing, and other less recognizable symptoms.

Some diagnostic tests such as the exercise stress test (ECG stress test) are less accurate for women, which may cause doctors to avoid using these tests. For instance, in young healthy women, the exercise stress test may give a false positive result. Routine treadmill tests may not pick up single-vessel heart disease, a more common type of CHD found in younger women. By delaying the diagnosis, the disease progresses untreated. Because women tend to develop and seek help for CHD later in life, diagnosis may also be hindered by the presence of other age-related diseases such as arthritis and osteoporosis.

Higher Death Rates in Women

When women do have heart attacks, they are more likely to die from them than men. One study published in the *New England Journal of Medicine* found that women had higher heart attack death rates during hospitalization (16.7 percent for women versus 11.5 percent for men). Since the advent of reperfusion strategies (opening the heart attack-related arteries), the mortality rates have declined for both men and women. Statistics from the National Heart, Lung, and Blood Institute and from the Framingham Heart Study reveal that more women who have heart attacks die within a year than men. This may be due, in part, to the fact that women tend to avoid or delay seeking medical attention for their symptoms, perhaps due to lack of awareness. Women also have heart attacks later in life. Age and the more advanced stage of CHD limit a woman's treatment options and may increase her risk of death.

Women may also die more often from heart attacks because they receive less aggressive aftercare than men. A recent national survey found that women are less likely than men to enroll in cardiac rehabilitation programs following a heart attack or bypass surgery. Those involved in cardiac rehab programs are more likely to receive treatment for CHD risk factors. It may be that women, who are trained in North American culture to be caregivers for others, are less willing to care for themselves.

Risk Factors for CHD in Women

Physiologically, men and women are different, so it shouldn't surprise us that CHD develops a bit differently in women and men. Some of the risk factors for CHD impact women differently than men.

Cigarette Smoking

An extensive twelve-year study in Norway recently published in the journal *Circulation* concluded that smoking poses greater dangers to women's hearts than to men's. Women who smoke twenty cigarettes or more per day are six times more likely to have a heart attack than women who never smoked. For men, the risk was 2.8 times greater when compared to nonsmoking males. Why the difference? Cigarette smoking targets two of women's "natural protectors"—estrogen and higher amounts of "good" HDL cholesterol circulating in the blood. Researchers speculate that cigarette smoking may cause an "antiestrogenic effect" and lower HDL more in women than in men.

Women who smoke and take birth control pills are at even greater risk. Taking birth control pills and smoking increase a woman's risk of heart attack by as much as 39 times compared with women who don't smoke or take birth control pills.

Increasing Age

Compared with men, women's risk of heart disease is relatively low until menopause. The female hormone estrogen may have a protective effect by raising a woman's "good" HDL cholesterol and lowering "bad" LDL cholesterol. However, after menopause and the subsequent decrease in estrogen, a woman's risk of heart attack rises. At age sixty-five, a woman's risk for heart attack is nearly that of men's.

Diabetes

Diabetes mellitus occurs when the body keeps too much glucose (sugar) in the bloodstream. The disease is a major risk factor for CHD and heart attack for both men and women, but it impacts women's risk even more dramatically. Having diabetes increases a woman's CHD risk by three to seven times compared with a twofold to threefold increase in men. This may be because diabetes in women has an especially negative effect on blood fats and blood pressure.

Cholesterol/Triglycerides

Total cholesterol levels are not as strong an indicator of heart disease for women as for men. For women, it appears that HDL levels are more important. Low levels of "good" HDL cholesterol are a reliable indicator of CHD in women. Low HDL levels appear to be a greater risk for CHD and heart attack for women older than sixty-five than in men of the same age. Some heart disease experts suggest that the national guideline of HDL levels of less than 35 mg/dL as an independent risk factor for CHD may be too low for women. They suggest 45 mg/dL or even higher HDL is a better standard.

In addition, women's trigylceride levels appear to have more influence in women's heart health. Women with trigylcerides higher than 190 mg/dL have a greater heart disease risk. Men's risk doesn't increase significantly until triglycerides reach 400 mg/dL.

Weight

Being overweight contributes to increased risks for CHD and heart attacks for both men and women. However, when women accumulate their extra pounds around the waist, they are more subject to high blood pressure and insulin resistance, a precursor to diabetes—both risk factors for CHD.

CHD and Hormone Replacement Therapy (HRT)

Estrogen is a female hormone made primarily by a woman's ovaries. Estrogen helps keep women's bones strong and protects against heart disease. As women approach menopause, their level of estrogen drops and their risk for heart attack and stroke rises slowly. Women who undergo *surgical menopause* (removal of the ovaries) and who don't take estrogen replacement experience a sharp rise in the risk of heart attack and stroke. (A woman who undergoes *partial hysterectomy*—removal of the uterus, leaving at least one ovary—retains her hormonal protection.)

For many years, women and their doctors believed that *hormone replacement therapy* or *HRT* (given in pills or patches that contain estrogen or the combination of hormones, estrogen-progestin) provided postmenopausal women with protection against heart disease and heart attacks. New research from the large-scale Heart and Estrogen Replacement Study (HERS) found that HRT provides no protective heart benefit for women with heart disease. Additionally, the Estrogen Replacement and Atherosclerosis (ERA) Trial found HRT did not slow the progression of atherosclerosis in women with heart disease or blood vessel disease.

The American Heart Association advises doctors against prescribing HRT for the sole purpose of preventing heart attacks and strokes in women with heart disease. Instead, they recommend women with heart disease reduce their risk of heart attack and stroke by making lifestyles changes such as quitting smoking, losing weight, and exercising regularly. These are considered first-line CHD therapies. Medications to reduce high cholesterol and/or high blood pressure can also help lower risk. There is evidence that statin medications, which lower cholesterol, are underprescribed in women and could help lower cholesterol levels better than hormone replacement therapy.

Population studies in the past have indicated that HRT reduces heart attacks in healthy women, those without evidence of heart disease. These studies are not definitive since the women were not randomly assigned to treatment. Also, women who participated in these studies were healthier, which may account for the lower incidence of heart attacks and strokes.

These new developments leave women and their doctors in a difficult place. HRT can be effective for decreasing the bone thinning of osteoporosis and for reducing menopausal hot flashes and vaginal dryness. However, HRT carries risks, too. Any woman, with or without established heart disease, who is considering HRT should talk with her doctor about the benefits and risks. Use the information below to help you and your doctor make the right choice for you.

Known and Potential Benefits of HRT

- HRT raises "good" HDL cholesterol and lowers "bad" LDL cholesterol. Skin patches may not have these benefits.
- The long-term Nurses' Health Study found that healthy women who took HRT had a lower risk of heart disease and death from most major diseases (except breast cancer).
- HRT keeps arteries flexible and increases blood flow, which makes them more able to respond to exercise and physical stress.
- HRT can help relieve menopausal symptoms such as hot flashes and help prevent bone loss.

Known and Potential Risks of HRT

- HRT does not reduce the risk of heart attack or dying from CHD in women who have heart disease.
- HRT using estrogen alone increases the risk of endometrial

and uterine cancers; combining estrogen and progestin helps reduce the risk.

- HRT increases the risk of gallbladder disease. Skin patches may not.
- It's unknown whether HRT increases breast cancer risk. Some studies show that it does; others show it does not.
- HRT raises triglyceride levels and possibly heart disease risk.
- Taking HRT when immobilized increases the risk for developing blood clots.
- Any woman who has the following conditions should be cautious about taking HRT:
  - liver disease (active or chronic)
  - history of breast or uterine cancer, or a family history of breast cancer
  - gallbladder disease
  - history of blood clots, especially in the arteries of the legs or lungs
  - CHD
  - obesity
  - diabetes
  - high blood pressure
  - history of stroke

Reducing Your Risk of CHD

If you're a woman with CHD or concerned about CHD, here's how you can reduce your risk:

Identify your risk factors. Work closely with your doctor to determine exactly what your heart disease risk factors are.

Reduce your risk factors. Lower your risk by making healthy lifestyle changes. Eat a low-fat, low-cholesterol diet. Lose excess weight. Lower your high cholesterol and your high blood pressure. Quit smoking and limit alcohol to no more than one drink per day. See chapter 9 for more information on heart-healthy lifestyle changes.

Talk with your doctor about HRT. Carefully weigh the risks and benefits of taking HRT, especially if you have established heart disease.

Know women's warning signs of heart attack. Too often, women don't recognize when they're having a heart attack. Women often have subtler symptoms. Recognizing heart attack symptoms can save your life.

Respond to warning signs. Don't wait if you think you may be having a heart attack. Call for emergency medical help (911 or other number) immediately. (See chapter 4 for more advice about responding to a heart attack.)

Less Typical Heart Attack / Heart Disease Symptoms Often Experienced by Women

- Chronic breathlessness or waking at night with difficulty breathing
- Overwhelming sense of doom, chronic fatigue
- Unexplained dizziness or blackouts
- Swelling, especially in the ankles and/or lower legs
- Rapid heartbeats
- Nausea or gastric upset

6 Getting a Diagnosis

Doctors today have a number of tests available to diagnose heart disease. The sooner your coronary heart disease is diagnosed, the sooner you can begin treatment to help prevent further atherosclerotic buildup (or in some cases, even reverse it) and help prevent a potentially deadly heart attack.

There is no single test for CHD. Diagnosing heart disease can be quite complicated because sometimes more than one type of heart disease occurs in the same person at the same time. Additionally, you may have other health problems that make it more difficult to determine exactly what's going on. To evaluate your heart health, your doctor has to be a bit of a detective. He or she will use a number of clues from a variety of sources to make a diagnosis. Your diagnosis will be based on:

- your medical history/interview
- a physical examination
- diagnostic tests

Your Medical History/Interview

The first thing your doctor will likely do is review your medical history and conduct a medical interview. Your medical history will include a number of questions about illnesses, surgeries, etc., that you or close family members have had. Providing complete and thorough information will help your doctor get a more accurate picture of your health. During the interview, your doctor will review your medical history with you and ask you a number of questions about your current state of health, including any symptoms you may be having. You should be prepared to answer questions such as:

- Have you or anyone in your family had a heart attack, stroke, or circulatory problem?
- What medications do you take?
- Have you ever had an abnormal electrocardiogram or exercise stress test?
- Have you ever taken heart medications or cholesterol-lowering medications?
- Describe your symptoms. When do these symptoms occur?
- What makes these symptoms better or worse?

Physical Examination

Once your doctor has thoroughly interviewed you about your medical history and your symptoms, he or she will conduct a physical exam. By listening, feeling, and observing specific areas of your body, your doctor can get clues about what's going on. This includes checking your vital signs—pulse, blood pressure, breath rate. If you have no CHD symptoms, your doctor may detect signs of poor circulation elsewhere in your body. Using a stethoscope, he or she will listen to your heart for irregular sounds and examine your neck, abdomen, and elsewhere for evidence of *bruits* or rough sounds produced by turbulent blood flow through narrowed arteries. Your doctor will also listen to your lungs, looking for signs of extra fluid buildup.

By carefully observing the veins in the neck while you're in various positions, the doctor can detect elevated pressures on the right side of the heart. He or she will also look for skin that is cool and pale or bluish (*cyanotic*), a sign of vascular disease. Since severe atherosclerosis in the legs can cause hair loss and thickening of the toenails, the doctor should carefully examine your feet and legs. The doctor will look for evidence of swelling (*edema*), especially in your feet, ankles, and legs.

Common Diagnostic Tests for CHD

- Blood tests (lipid profile, blood count, chemistries)
- Electrocardiography (ECG or EKG)
- Chest X-ray
- Nuclear scanning and stress testing
- Catheterization and angiography
- Advanced imaging (CT, SPECT, MUGA, PET, MRI)

Standard Diagnostic Tests

The diagnostic tests your doctor uses will depend on your symptoms, your medical history, your risk factors, and the results of your physical exam. The specific diagnostic tests selected will be tailored for you. If your history, symptoms, and physical examination don't indicate problems, your doctor will likely order only a few tests. Regardless of whether or not you have CHD symptoms, you'll probably need more than one diagnostic test because different tests provide the doctor with different information. Fortunately, many of the tests for CHD are *noninvasive*—they're done outside the body and are painless.

An electrocardiogram (ECG or EKG) reflects the overall health of the heart muscle and whether it's beating normally. The test does not tell whether arteries are blocked.

Electrocardiography (ECG or EKG)

One of the most common tests for heart disease, *electrocardiography (ECG)* records the electrical activity of the heart. ECGs are also called EKGs. Your doctor will likely order an ECG if you have CHD symptoms such as chest pain, shortness of breath, palpitations (rapid fluttering of the heart), or fainting. Some doctors like to do an ECG on anyone over age forty during routine examinations.

The ECG is painless and takes less than ten minutes. You'll lie on an examination table while a doctor, nurse, or technician attaches twelve small disks, electrodes, at various points on your body. These electrodes are attached to wires, which are attaching to the electrocardiogram machine; then you lie quietly while these electrodes pick up the electrical impulses of your heart. As the machine records your heart's activity, the results are recorded as "waves" displayed on a monitor or printed on paper.

The ECG provides valuable information about your heart's rate, rhythm, whether you've previously had a heart attack, or have structural abnormalities. However, like most tests, it's not without limitations. A normal ECG doesn't rule out CHD. In fact, you may have a totally normal resting ECG but still have a 90 percent narrowing of a major coronary artery. Unfortunately, changes in ECG results often don't occur until atherosclerosis is very severe or after structural damage has occurred.

Likewise, an abnormal ECG doesn't mean you definitely have CHD, particularly if you don't have CHD symptoms or risk factors. ECG abnormalities can be caused by non-heart problems such as blood/tissue salt (electrolyte) abnormalities, lung disease, and some types of medication.

Exercise Stress Test

The *exercise stress test* is a recording of your heart's electrical activity under stress. It's also referred to as a *stress ECG* or a *treadmill test*. It's usually done while you're walking on a treadmill or pedaling a stationary bike. Because the stress test produces higher heart rates than the resting ECG, it's better able to detect problems such as poor circulation and insufficient blood and oxygen supply in the coronary arteries. The test is an excellent measure of how your heart muscle functions.

The exercise test can also detect exercise-related heart rhythm disturbances and abnormalities in blood pressure response. If you've had a heart attack or you're already being treated for heart problems with medications, your doctor may order periodic stress ECG tests to check on the severity of the coronary artery obstruction and to monitor your progress. The test also can be used to design an exercise program to strengthen your heart.

If your doctor orders an exercise stress test for you:

- Plan for the test to take about an hour. You'll be asked to walk or pedal for five to fifteen minutes. The rest of the time you'll be monitored at rest.
- Eat only a light breakfast or lunch before taking the test. Allow at least two hours between your meal and your exercise stress test.
- Take your medications as usual, unless directed otherwise. Some people need to stop taking their medications a day or two before the test—your doctor will tell you if that's necessary. (Some tests are designed to detect a problem and medications are withheld. Other tests are to see how well the person is protected with medications.)
- Wear comfortable clothing and walking shoes.
- Let the doctor, nurse, or technician know immediately if you feel chest discomfort or shortness of breath during the test.

For most people, undergoing an exercise stress test is perfectly safe. Since the test stresses the heart, there is a small risk of suffering a heart attack or serious rhythm disturbance, but the risk is very slight. Your doctor, nurses, and the technicians on hand are trained to handle any type of heart emergency that might occur.

The exercise stress test isn't for everyone. Some people cannot walk on a treadmill. Some have uninterpretable results that require a different type of stress test. An exercise stress test is *not* for you if you have:

- chest pain (angina) at rest
- potentially life-threatening heart rhythm problems (arrhythmias)
- infection, inflammation, or swelling of the heart sac (pericarditis), heart muscle (myocarditis), or heart valves (endocarditis)
- tear on the inner lining of the aorta (aortic dissection)
- blood clots in the lungs (pulmonary infarct or embolus)
- other serious or acute illness

The exercise stress test is a fairly reliable test for detecting severe coronary blockages of the main artery or blockages of all three major coronary vessels (at least 50 percent narrowed). However, it's not perfect. It will detect obstructive CHD in about 67 percent of those with the disease in one of the three major arteries. When the test is negative, it does not give any information about the presence or absence of plaque. Your doctor will interpret the results of your exercise test in concert with your symptoms, your medical history, your risk factors, and other test results.

Ambulatory ECG (Holter Monitoring)

A variation on the exercise stress test, an *ambulatory ECG*, (also called *Holter monitoring* for its inventor), monitors the heart continuously during a twenty-four hour period. This test can help detect heart problems that seem to come and go. If you under go this test, several electrodes will be attached to your chest so that a portable recording device, about the size of an audio cassette player, can record your heart's electrical activity. It can detect abnormal heart rhythms and changes related to lack of blood flow. You keep the device on for a twenty-four-hour period, even when you're sleeping. The doctor will also likely ask you to keep an activity diary, which can be compared with the test results to verify if the symptoms correspond with the ECG abnormalities.

Chest X-ray

Your doctor may order a chest X-ray to look at the size and shape of your heart and major blood vessels. A chest X-ray also lets the doctor examine your lungs. If your heart isn't pumping strongly enough, for instance, fluid may leak into the air sacs of the lungs (*pulmonary edema*).

A chest X-ray is quick and painless. You'll be asked to remove your clothing and jewelry from the waist up and put on a hospital gown. You'll stand against a plate that holds the X-ray film with your arms held up or out to the sides. You'll be asked to take a breath and hold it, which helps the heart and lungs appear on the X-ray.

Having a chest X-ray with today's low-dose machines is quite safe. However, if you're pregnant, be sure to tell your doctor before having a chest X-ray. Risk to the baby is low, but special precautions should be taken to protect the baby from exposure. A chest X-ray during pregnancy is done only when absolutely necessary.

Echocardiography

Perhaps you've heard of an *echocardiogram*. This noninvasive technology, *echocardiography*, uses high-pitched sound waves (*ultrasound*) directed toward your heart to reflect back a "picture" of the heart. Ultrasound uses the same principles that bats or submarines use to navigate. Echocardiography provides precise information about your heart's function, its valves, and adjacent structures.

One type of ultrasound, the Doppler, detects heart sounds and displays an image of the blood flowing between different chambers of the heart. A color map and other precise measurements can be made with the Doppler ultrasound to assess the severity of narrowing or leakage in one or more heart valves. It can also measure the pressure inside the lungs.

Your echocardiogram is usually done in the cardiologist's office or laboratory (or in the hospital if you're hospitalized). You don't have to follow any special instructions before having the test. You'll be asked to remove your clothing from the waist up and put on a hospital gown or drape. You'll lie down on your back or left side. After having a special gel applied to your chest (the gel improves the transmission of ultrasound waves), the doctor, nurse, or lab technician will move a hand-held instrument (a *transducer*) over your chest. The transducer is attached to a monitoring screen and other components. The examination is painless and will take fifteen to thirty minutes. There is no known risk to having an ultrasound.

Certain conditions make it difficult to get a clear ultrasound image. Such conditions include:

- having lung disease (such as emphysema)
- being very overweight
- having spinal or chest wall abnormalities
- having very large breasts or breast implants
- having had chest or heart surgery or a chest injury
- if you're on a ventilator

Sometimes doctors use echocardiography to view the heart under stress with a *stress echocardiogram*. This test includes a

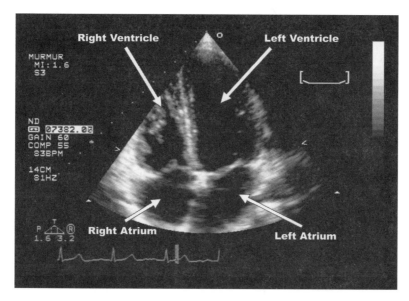

During an echocardiogram, sound waves produce an image of the beating heart. The test measures heart function and can detect narrowing arteries when combined with stress testing.

number of steps. First, your doctor will perform a resting echocardiogram. Next, you might be asked to walk on a treadmill, ride a stationary bike, or be given a medication, dobutamine, injected intravenously, which causes the heart to beat faster and stronger for a few minutes. Immediately after the exercise or medication has elevated your heart rate to a certain level, another echocardiogram is taken and the ultrasound images are captured on videotape or as a digital recording. This enables doctors to compare ultrasound images of the heart both at rest and under stress. A stress echocardiogram is slightly less accurate than nuclear scanning (see below) for detecting obstructive narrowing, but more accurate than an ECG stress test.

If you are scheduled for a stress echocardiogram, you may be asked to refrain from eating or drinking for several hours before the test. It's a good idea to ask your doctor if it's okay to take your routine medications, including prescriptions, over-the-counter medications, and herbal supplements, on the day of the test.

A specialized type of echocardiogram is the *transesophageal echocardiogram* (TEE). It magnifies the heart's structures (including the valves) and can detect blood clots that are hiding in the left atrium (top left chamber of the heart). These hidden clots can travel and may cause a stroke. TEE is also used in people during open-heart surgery to check the valves and heart muscle function. Unlike other forms of echocardiography, TEE is somewhat invasive. The test takes approximately twenty minutes and is usually done on an outpatient basis. The throat is numbed with a local anesthesia and a tube is passed through the esophagus, which lies directly behind the heart. The tube contains a tiny ultrasound crystal that reflects back the ultrasound image.

Nuclear Scans

Several types of nuclear scans are available to help doctors determine whether the heart is receiving enough blood flow under stress. Depending on the type of scan selected, nuclear scanning can tell the doctor about the size of the chambers of the heart, how the ventricles are pumping blood, and the level of blood flow to the heart muscle and lungs. Additionally, the doctor may order nuclear scans to monitor the effectiveness of medication or to measure improvement in blood flow to the heart following angioplasty or bypass surgery.

A blockage must be fairly severe—at least 50 percent blocked—before it can be detected with nuclear scanning. Scans can detect

On the left, a nuclear stress test shows normal blood flow at rest. The photo on the right shows where there is a lack of blood flow during exercise.

narrowing in 88 to 90 percent of people with serious blockages. A negative test can rule out severe obstructions in most people, but it doesn't eliminate the possibility of severe plaque in the arteries.

Nuclear Stress Test

The nuclear stress test provides your doctor with information about how well your heart is working and whether your heart has sustained any muscle damage. Nuclear stress tests can also determine whether arteries are narrowed. This test is similar to an exercise stress test, in which you walk on a treadmill or pedal a stationary bicycle. For this test you'll be given an injection of a radioactive material, called an *isotope*, just before you complete the exercise task. Next, you will lie on a table and a specialized camera will pass over your chest, taking images of your heart. The isotope gives off tiny amounts of radiation, which are detected by the camera, making it possible for doctors to observe the heart function.

Some people are alarmed by the idea of having radioactive material injected into their bodies. However, the amount of radiation you'll be exposed to is very small and safe. The benefits of the tests outweigh the small risk. If you're pregnant or possibly pregnant, you should avoid nuclear tests.

Single Photon Emission Computed Tomography (SPECT)

Another test that uses nuclear technology is the *single photon emission computed tomography (SPECT).* One of the most widely used tests, it shows how well blood flows to the heart muscle and how well the heart muscle is functioning in different regions. For this test, you'll be given an injection of a radioactive tracer, which allows doctors to see the blood flowing into your heart. While you're lying on a table, a machine will pass over your chest area as it takes images. Once the images are captured, a sophisticated computer "slices" the images, giving precise pictures that enable the doctor to see blood flow problems, both at rest and during exercise.

Multi-Unit Gated Acquisition (MUGA)

The *multi-unit gated acquisition (MUGA)* is another nuclear test which uses a radioactive isotope to show doctors whether areas of the heart have been damaged by previous heart attack or are deprived of circulation. It is used to assess heart muscle function at rest and under stress. For a resting stress test, you'll be given an injection of a radioactive isotope and asked to lie on a special table; a camera will take images of your heart. If you're taking a stress test, you'll be moved to another table, which has pedals at the end of it. You'll be asked to lie on the table and pedal as if you are riding a bicycle. As you're pedaling, images will be taken of your heart. This test also tells how effectively blood is being pumped from the lower chambers of your heart.

Advanced Imaging Diagnostic Tests

Recent developments in technology have allowed for even more sophisticated imaging of the heart and may enable doctors to diagnose CHD before a person has symptoms.

Standard Cardiac Computed Tomography (CT)

X-ray computed tomography (also known as a *CT* or *CAT scan*) produces cross-sectional images of the chest, including the heart, lungs, and major blood vessels. This scan is especially helpful in evaluating diseases of the large blood vessels, masses or tumors in the heart, and diseases of the heart sac or *pericardium*. It's also helpful in diagnosing blood clots on the lung or tears of the aorta.

The images are produced as an X-ray beam passes through the body. Unlike a regular X-ray machine, the CT X-ray machine rotates rapidly around the body. This allows images to be captured from various angles. A computer then combines the images and produces a detailed cross section of the body. Though there is a small amount of exposure to radiation, all CT scans are painless and involve little risk.

Coronary Calcium Scoring

A newer procedure, *coronary calcium scoring*, also called *cardiac CT for calcium scoring*, is a specialized type of CT scan that can help determine whether you have plaque in your arteries. In many instances, it can diagnose atherosclerosis before blockages become severe. Coronary calcium scoring is to heart disease what the mammogram is to breast cancer—an early-detection test.

With this advanced imaging technology, doctors are able to detect calcium in the arteries. Calcium itself does not cause a heart attack, but its presence is an important indicator of CHD and may predict heart attack risk. In the plaque building of atherosclerosis, the blood vessel walls are continually being injured and the body is constantly attempting to heal the injuries. As the body tries to repair the damaged area, calcium is deposited in the injured area. On routine X-rays, this hard calcium shows up only at a very late stage. With coronary calcium scoring, calcium deposits can be detected and measured at a very early stage. In fact, calcium scoring can determine the presence of CHD even when the arteries are less than 50 percent narrowed, something that many standard cardiac diagnostic tests are unable to do.

This screening study may be recommended if you have risk factors for CHD but no symptoms yet. People who are likely candidates for coronary calcium scoring include:

- men age 45 and older and women age 55 and older
- women who are postmenopausal
- people with a family history of heart disease
- past or present smokers
- people who have a sedentary lifestyle

- people who have a stressful lifestyle
- people with diabetes
- people with high blood pressure
- people with high LDL cholesterol or low HDL cholesterol
- people who are overweight or obese
- people who suffer from other vascular disease (such as carotid artery narrowing)

Note: If you're pregnant or think you might be pregnant, inform your doctor before having the test. It should be postponed until after delivery.

A coronary calcium scoring test doesn't require any special preparation, although you may be asked to avoid caffeine and smoking for about four hours prior to the test. If your heartbeat is rapid, you may be given a drug to slow the rate. Performed in the same manner as a standard CT scan, coronary calcium scoring is quick, painless, and involves minimal risk. The results of the test—your calcium score—indicate the amount of calcification in your arteries. The results may be listed as:

- no evidence of plaque
- minimal evidence of plaque
- mild evidence of plaque
- moderate evidence of plaque
- extensive evidence of plaque

Although coronary calcium scoring can be an indication of your risk for CHD, it has limitations. For instance, calcium deposits

A noninvasive diagnostic test, the 64-slice CTA scan provides a high-resolution image of the heart, helping doctors determine whether any narrowing in the arteries has occurred.

don't always signify a blockage in the arteries, and not all blockages contain calcium. In addition, the test is unable to detect soft plaque, the earliest form of artherosclerosis.

Some of the earlier technologies designed to detect calcium in the arteries have been proven to be less accurate than current scanners. Diagnostic tools such as the electron beam tomography (EBT), also called electron beam computed tomography (EBCT) has been replaced by the 64-Slice CT scanner to detect calcium. Similarly, electronic beam angiography (EBA) has been replaced by a CTA or CT angiography using the 64-Slice CT scanner (see below).

64-Slice Computed Coronary Angiography

One of the most promising new advances in CT scanning is the 64-Slice *Computed Coronary Angiography (CTA)*. This device is able to take nearly 200 images of the heart per second, far faster than standard CT scanners. The speed of the 64-Slice CT scanner allows it to virtually "freeze" motion images of the heart and arteries. Doctors can see exactly where blood flows within the arteries and determine whether there's a blockage. Thanks to the extremely high resolution of the images, results are more accurate than with a standard CT scan. When results of a 64-Slice CT scan show no blockages in the arteries, it reduces the need for more invasive diagnostic procedures, such as catheterization and angiography, both of which are explained later in this chapter.

This quick, painless procedure may involve placing a small IV in the arm to administer a contrast material (X-ray dye) to improve the view of the heart and arteries. You may be given a medication to slow your heartbeat so the motion of your heart is reduced. Once the scan begins, you'll be asked to hold your breath for only a few seconds, as opposed to the twenty-five to forty seconds normally required for standard CT scans. The procedure poses little risk other than a small amount of radiation and the occasional side effects associated with the (X-ray dye).

Despite its many benefits, this imaging technique isn't recommended for everyone. Certain situations can reduce the accuracy of the test or can make it difficult to see inside the arteries. Such situations include calcification in the arteries (a common development if you have CHD), having a stent in an artery, and having a metal heart valve.

Cardiac Positron-Emission Tomography (PET)

A *cardiac positron-emission tomography (PET)* scan is a high-tech nuclear scan. For a PET scan, you're asked to remove your clothes above the waist and lie on a scanning table, which slides through a large tube-like machine—the PET scanner. Computerized pictures of your heart will be taken while it's at work. Doctors can measure blood flow and metabolism (inner workings of cells) in the heart. This part of the test takes ten to fifteen minutes. Then, you'll be given an injection of a radioactive tracer; after about forty-five minutes, after the tracer has circulated into the bloodstream, more pictures will be taken.

This technology is a very accurate, noninvasive way to detect CHD. It can also identify injured heart tissue. The widespread use of PET has been limited, in part because it's expensive.

Magnetic Resonance Imaging (MRI)

Unlike other scans, which use X-ray technology, *magnetic resonance imaging (MRI)* uses powerful magnets and radio waves to produce clear, three-dimensional images of the heart's chambers and large vessels without having to use X-ray contrast agents (dyes). In addition, adjacent bone and air doesn't interfere with the images. An MRI gives your doctor a look at your heart muscle and helps determine whether you've suffered any damage to your heart muscle from a heart attack. The test can also evaluate diseases of the larger blood vessels. Cardiac MRI may also prove to be a tool that shows blood flow problems and blockages in the coronary arteries, especially for those, such as patients with kidney disease, who can't tolerate X-ray dye.

There are no known risks from using MRI. However, because MRI depends on magnetic forces, if you have a pacemaker or other metal in the body, you can't undergo the test.

Cardiac Catheterization and Angiography

Also called *coronary angiography*, *arteriography*, or *angiocardiography*, this diagnostic technique shows blood flow problems and blockages in the coronary arteries. It can measure blood pressure in the heart, determine how much oxygen is in the blood, and provide information about the structure and function of the heart muscle, heart valves, and arteries. Because techniques have become so refined, you may be able to have a therapeutic procedure (angioplasty or stenting) immediately following this diagnostic procedure. (See chapter 8 for more information on angioplasty and stenting.)

During cardiac catheterization and angiography, a long, sterile, flexible tube called a *catheter* is threaded through an artery in the leg or arm up into the heart. Then a liquid contrast material (X-ray dye) is injected into the tube. The contrast material allows the heart and blood vessels to show up on an X-ray monitor in a digital picture called an *angiogram* or *arteriogram*.

Your doctor may order cardiac catheterization and angiography as a diagnostic tool if:

- he or she suspects you have significant CHD

- you'll be undergoing heart surgery such as bypass surgery
- you have heart valve problems, including valve narrowing (stenosis) or blood backflow through an abnormal valve (called insufficiency or regurgitation)
- he or she suspects you have heart muscle damage (cardiomyopathy)

Cardiac catheterization and angiography is done in a special *catheterization laboratory ("cath" lab)* in a hospital.

Preparing for Cardiac Catheterization

- Don't eat or drink anything after midnight the night before the procedure (except small amounts of water for taking medication). If catheterization is scheduled for the afternoon, your doctor may allow you to have clear liquids for breakfast.
- Empty your bladder before the exam.
- Leave jewelry at home.
- Inform your doctor if you're allergic to X-ray dye. Most hospitals use the newer X-ray dyes, which decrease (but do not totally eliminate) allergic reactions. Doctors pretreat those who have dye allergies with antihistamines and corticosteroids to reduce the likelihood of an allergic reaction.
- If you're pregnant, be sure to let your doctor know.

The area on your leg or arm where the catheter will be inserted will be cleaned and shaved. An intravenous line will be inserted into your arm to deliver fluids and medications. Then you'll be taken to the cath lab and placed on a flat table under an X-ray machine. The nurses will attach electrocardiogram electrodes to your arms and legs, and you'll be given medication to help you relax. A blood pressure cuff will be put on your arm, and a *pulse oximeter* (a noninvasive, clothespin-like monitor for blood oxygen content) will be placed on your finger.

You usually won't be totally asleep during the procedure, but you may doze. The cardiologist and other members of your cath team will likely explain what's being done throughout the process and let you know what sensations to expect. The doctor numbs the insertion site, usually the area over the femoral artery located in the groin. An artery at the wrist or at the inside elbow may be used, especially if leg arteries have severe blockages. The cardiologist inserts a needle into the vessel, and then threads a thin guide wire through the needle. After withdrawing the needle, the doctor inserts a flexible tube called a *sheath* into the blood vessel over the guide wire. The sheath has a one-way valve that allows the catheter to be inserted, but keeps blood from leaking out.

In rare cases, an incision is made to access the artery. This technique, known as a *cutdown*, was more common in the past. It takes a little longer and requires stitches to repair the incision.

By watching the X-ray video carefully to monitor the progress, the doctor advances the catheter through the blood vessels to your heart. During the procedure, the cardiologist may insert several catheters via the same entry site into various parts of your heart. You will not feel the catheter when it's inside. Once in the heart, the catheter(s) can perform functions such as measuring the pressure in the chambers, taking blood samples, and injecting X-ray dye (also called contrast) for an angiogram (pictures of arteries). When contrast material is injected into the main pumping chamber of the heart or into the main artery, you'll feel a hot sensation that lasts for five to twenty seconds. It's important to remain very still so that the X-ray images will be clear. You may also feel your heart "skip beats." Occasionally, you may feel nauseated or hot all over during the procedure, which usually passes after a minute or so. These are all normal sensations and shouldn't alarm you. However, let the doctor know when you experience these feelings or if you feel any chest pain.

Follow-up to Cardiac Catheterization

After all the tests and procedures are completed, the catheter(s) will be removed. The insertion site will be compressed or the cardiologist will insert a closure device. About twenty minutes of compression allows the body to make its own blood clot to seal the opening. A specialized pressure dressing may then be applied to the wound to help prevent bleeding. After the catheterization, you'll be required to lie flat on your back for six to eight hours with your arm or leg extended. During this time, the cath nurse will monitor your vital signs and keep an eye on the catheter insertion site to make sure it's not bleeding. He or she will also monitor the pulse, color, and temperature of the arm or leg used for the procedure. Let the nurse know if you notice any swelling, bleeding, or pain where the catheter was inserted. If your doctor used a closure device (stitches, plugs, or a type of sealer) on the insertion site, the required bed rest time is much shorter—as little as an hour. Once you've recovered sufficiently and no critical blockages are present, the doctor will release you to go home.

Before leaving the clinic or hospital, you should:

- Ask about results. You can usually talk with your doctor about your condition right after the procedure. Your doctor will likely come into the recovery room and talk with you about your results. He or she will also let your family know the results right after the procedure.
- Ask the doctor when you can resume eating and drinking.
- Have someone available to drive you home. You shouldn't drive for at least twenty-four hours following the procedure.

When you return home you should:

- Avoid strenuous activity for at least forty-eight hours after the procedure.
- Call the doctor's office immediately if the catheter insertion site becomes swollen, red, painful, or oozes blood, or if the limb becomes painful, cold and pale, or has a weak or absent pulse.
- Return to the doctor's office for follow-up within five to seven days.

Risks of Cardiac Catheterization

While cardiac catheterization and angiography can provide your doctor with valuable information about your heart's health, it's not without risk. In most cases, the procedure is safe. However, serious complications are possible, including death, stroke or heart attack, abnormal heartbeat (arrhythmia), puncture of a blood vessel or the heart muscle, bleeding, blood clotting or infection at the site of insertion, a blocked blood vessel in the arm or leg where the catheter was inserted, or an allergic reaction to the X-ray dye. Keep in mind that serious complications are rare. They usually occur in people who are critically ill or when catheterization is done under emergency conditions. You're at greater risk for serious complications if you have chronic illnesses such as kidney failure, insulin-dependent diabetes, severe lung disease, severely decreased heart function, or if you're older than eighty years of age. If you have kidney problems, you're at greater risk for dye-related kidney complications. Your cath team will need to take special precautions to minimize your risk and avoid problems.

After a Diagnosis of CHD: Coping Emotionally

If your diagnostic tests indicate that you have CHD, realize that it can have an emotional impact on you. It's easy to think of CHD as a purely physical disease. However, the diagnosis of heart disease is bound to affect you emotionally. In fact, depression is a very common response to the diagnosis of CHD or following a heart attack or heart surgery. It's often triggered by feelings of loss—perhaps loss of the way your body once was or loss of the old, familiar lifestyle. Or it may be triggered by fears—of dying, of having another heart attack, or of feeling vulnerable and frail. If you find yourself unable to sleep, tearful, or having feelings of hopelessness and despair, talk with your doctor. He or she can provide treatment for your symptoms of depression.

Following are some strategies for dealing with depression, anxiety, or fears about your heart disease:

Communicate with your doctor. Be sure to talk openly with

your doctor about your condition and your emotions. If you have questions or concerns, don't wait for a scheduled appointment; call the doctor. If your doctor doesn't make him or herself available to you, or you don't feel comfortable talking with them, find a new doctor.

Become empowered. By making the appropriate lifestyle changes and taking your medications, you can take control of your disease rather than letting it take control of you.

Avoid denial. Don't block out your physical problem hoping it will "just go away."

Don't deny your emotions. Allow yourself to feel your feelings deeply. Acknowledge that having heart disease is an emotionally painful condition.

Avoid withdrawal. Don't wall yourself off from others. Stay involved with family, friends, and colleagues.

Talk to others. Call friends or close family members and talk about how you feel. Set yourself a goal to talk to someone for at least a few minutes every day. Join a group. There are support groups for cardiac patients. Ask your doctor for a referral.

Get out. You may have to force yourself to go out at first, but do it. Accept a variety of invitations.

Keep a journal. Just writing down how you feel can help. When you've finished writing down all your negative feelings, start a new page with the heading "Things I'm Doing for Myself Today."

7 Medications for Coronary Heart Disease

Once your doctor has confirmed that you have coronary heart disease, undoubtedly your next question is "What do I do about it?" Your treatment will depend on the severity of your CHD and your general health. CHD treatment aims to prevent or reverse significant artery narrowing, make sure your heart gets enough oxygen to prevent heart attacks, and protect your heart from being damaged. Medications can help.

A number of medications have proven effective in treating CHD. For many people, drug therapy can help prevent a heart attack or stroke. It can also help prevent complications and slow the progression of atherosclerosis. Unlike surgical options, heart medications aren't invasive. They're also less expensive.

All drugs, however, have side effects. Some of these are minor; others are more serious. For anyone taking medication, the benefits of the medication must be weighed against the risks. That's why it's important that you only take heart medication under the direction and close supervision of your doctor.

Common CHD Medications

A number of medications are used to prevent and/or treat CHD. Your doctor may prescribe one or a combination of medications for you, depending on the nature of your CHD and other health problems. Medications for CHD include the following:

Anti-Anginal Medications

Nitrates

Often prescribed to relieve angina, *nitrates*—usually nitroglycerine—widen the coronary arteries. This increases blood flow to the heart. They also dilate the veins, which slows the return of blood to the heart and makes the heart work less.

If you have severe angina, your doctor may prescribe nitroglycerine (NTG) tablets or a spray that you put under your tongue. Nitroglycerine works very fast to relieve pain. If you need daily doses of nitrate medication, your doctor may prescribe it in a capsule by mouth or as a cream or patch that's placed on the skin. Even if you take long-acting preparations (pills or patches), you may still need to take nitrate tablets or spray, as needed, if breakthrough pain occurs. Intravenous NTG is available for patients who are hospitalized.

The most problematic side effect of nitrate medication is a sudden drop in blood pressure when you stand from sitting or lying down (*orthostatic hypotension*). If your systolic blood pressure is below 90 mmHg, nitroglycerine probably isn't a good choice. The medication can also cause flushing, headache, dizziness, and rapid heartbeat (*tachycardia*). Some side effects, such as headache, usually lessen after taking the medication for several days.

In rare cases, topical nitrates can cause a skin rash. Alcohol may worsen side effects.

A note of caution: Never take nitroglycerine if you've been taking sildenafil (Viagra), bardenafil (*Levitra*), or tadalafil (*Cialis*). It can cause a life-threatening drop in blood pressure. If you've been taking one of these medications and you're having chest pain—even severe chest pain—*don't* take nitroglycerine. Instead, go to the hospital immediately.

All forms of nitrates have a limited shelf life. Nitrates that are too old simply won't work. Talk with your pharmacist about how long your nitrates will be effective and how to store them to keep them at their peak.

Commonly prescribed nitrates: nitroglycerine (*NTG, Nitro-Bid, Nitrostat, Nitrogard*). Longer-acting preparations are isosorbide mononitrate or dinitrate (*ISMO, Monoket, Imdur, Sorbitrate, Isordil*)

Beta-Blockers

Beta-blockers are another type of drug commonly prescribed for angina. Beta-blockers decrease heart rate, reduce the strength of the heart's contractions, and lower blood pressure. As a result, they decrease the heart's need for oxygen. When you drive your car at fifty miles per hour instead of eighty miles per hour, you use less gas. The same principle applies to the heart. The slower the heart rate, the less fuel or oxygen the heart needs. Beta-blockers can also help normalize some types of heart rhythm disturbances (abnormal beats). Additionally, this medication has been proven to decrease sudden death in people after a heart attack and to reduce the severity of a heart attack when given immediately.

Beta-blockers can also have a number of side effects, such as wheezing and breathlessness in people with asthma. If you have coronary spasm, beta-blockers can worsen your angina. Abruptly stopping beta-blockers may cause an increase in heart rate and blood pressure. In some cases, beta-blockers worsen heart failure acutely. Other side effects include fatigue, dizziness, depression, diarrhea, skin rash, and sexual dysfunction. However, long term, beta-blockers have been proven to improve symptoms and de-crease mortality in people with heart failure.

Commonly prescribed beta-blockers: atenolol (*Tenormin*), metoprolol (*Lopressor, Toprol XL*), nadolol (*Corgard*), propranolol (*Inderal*), and carvedilol (*Coreg*)

Calcium Channel Blockers

As the name implies, *calcium channel blockers* block or inhibit the movement of calcium in the heart, nerves, and blood vessel walls. These drugs reduce blood pressure and dilate coronary ar-teries, making them useful in treating angina (including the type caused by spasm). They also normalize some types of arrhythmias. People who aren't helped by or can't take nitroglycerine or beta-blockers can often get relief using calcium channel blockers.

If you're taking calcium channel blockers, avoid drinking grapefruit juice at the time you take the medication. Grapefruit juice contains a component that interferes with the liver's ability to clear certain drugs, such as nifedipine (*Adalat, Procardia*), felo-dipine (*Plendil*), and nimodipine (*Nimotop*). Drinking grapefruit juice and taking these drugs can allow toxic levels of the drugs to build up in the blood.

Commonly prescribed calcium channel blockers: diltiazem hy-drochloride (*Cardizem, Dilacor, Cartia XT*), amlodipine (*Norvasc*), felodipine (*Plendil*), nimodipine (*Nimotop*), nifedipine (*Adalat, Procardia*), nicardipine (*Cardene*), and verapamil (*Calan, Isoptin, Verelan, Covera*)

Ranolazine (Ranexa)

A newer anti-anginal medication, *ranolazine (Ranexa)* works by an as yet unknown mechanism. Most people taking this drug find they have an increased tolerance for exercise and the ability to exercise for longer periods of time before experiencing symptoms of angina. Designed to treat chronic stable angina, ranolazine may be recommended if nitrates, beta-blockers, and calcium channel blockers haven't provided complete relief of your symptoms. In some cases, doctors may prescribe ranolazine in combination with other anti-anginal medications to provide additional relief. The drug isn't recommended, however, during an acute angina attack. Since drug interactions are common, always discuss possible side effects with your doctor.

Because Ranexa can cause side effects that impair your reactions and your thinking, be careful if you drive when taking the drug. Other side effects include dizziness, headache, blurred vision, dry mouth, nausea, vomiting, stomach pain, constipation, weakness, and ringing in your ears. As with calcium channel blockers, you should avoid drinking grapefruit juice if you're taking Ranexa.

Blood Thinners

The body defends itself against bleeding to death by forming blood clots. However, blood's tendency to clot in the coronary arteries can also cause angina and heart attacks. There are two major ways that blood clots:

- Platelets (tiny cells circulating in the bloodstream) stick to damaged surfaces and to one another to form a so-called white clot (*white thrombus*).
- Specialized blood proteins are activated and form a gel-like red ball or red clot (*red thrombus*).

Blood thinners work to alter one or both of these blood-clotting mechanisms.

Antiplatelet Agents

These drugs reduce the blood's ability to clot by inhibiting the normal functioning of platelets. Aspirin is one of the best-known antiplatelet medications. It helps prevent blood clot formation on existing plaque, which reduces the risk of heart attacks. Over time, aspirin makes the blood more resistant to forming clots. Aspirin is usually prescribed to all patients with CHD, unless they have an allergy or other problem. It's the first medication that's given in an emergency room during a heart attack. It's also used after coronary angioplasty and stenting to prevent blood clots and help prolong the lifespan of bypasses created during coronary bypass surgery. (See chapter 8 for more information on these procedures.)

Thienopyridines—clopidogrel (*Plavix*) and ticlopidine (*Ticlid*)—are stronger than aspirin and are used with aspirin after coronary stenting to prevent a clot from forming in the stent. In the past, these drugs were prescribed for a period of one month after a person had a noncoated or bare metal stent (BMS) placed. However, it has since been determined that there is a benefit in continuing clopidogrel for up to one year after the placement of a stent. Some patients may need to take them longer, especially if they had a coronary event despite taking aspirin.

For people who receive intracoronary radiation (also called *brachytherapy*) for recurrent blockages, the prescription for these blood thinners is usually for a minimum of twelve months; this drug is often prescribed in addition to aspirin.

Clopidogrel is the drug of choice because of its low rate of side effects. Ticlopidine is only used if the person has an allergy to clopidogrel (rare). Taking ticlopidine requires blood testing every two weeks to monitor for severe reductions in white blood cell count. This drug is also more likely to cause a rash. Other drugs are being developed.

The most potent available antiplatelet drugs are intravenous *glycoprotein llb/llla antagonists* including abciximab (*ReoPro*), eptifibatide (*Integrilin*), and tirofiban (*Aggrastat*). They are only given in the hospital to people who have unstable angina or a heart attack, or during angioplasty and stenting. They can dramatically improve the treatment outcomes for people who have unstable angina and for higher-risk patients in cath labs.

Commonly prescribed antiplatelet agents: aspirin and clopidogrel (*Plavix*)

Anticoagulants

These blood-thinning drugs inhibit the specialized blood proteins that form a red blood clot (red thrombus). They are often given during and after a heart attack to prevent clots from forming. Your doctor may also prescribe an anticoagulant medication if you have atrial fibrillation (a type of irregular heartbeat) or an artificial heart valve. These drugs don't dissolve existing blood clots. They can, however, prevent new clots from forming or prevent existing clots from getting bigger. They can be administered both intravenously and by mouth.

The most common oral anticoagulant is warfarin (*Coumadin*), which interferes with blood clotting by blocking the body's use of vitamin K. The drug takes two to three days to start working and a similar amount of time to stop working. Dosage varies greatly from person to person. If you take warfarin, you'll need to have your blood checked regularly to ensure the dosage is right for you. If the dose is too little, the blood will be too thick and clotting may occur. If the dose is too much, the blood will be too thin and there's a risk of bleeding complications.

A number of drugs—antibiotics, steroids, diuretics, antidepressants, and pain relievers, among others—can interact with warfarin and cause serious complications. It's important to consult your doctor any time a new medication is prescribed for you. The drug can be used long term for valve problems, some heart rhythm disturbances (atrial fibrillation), and for some people with CHD. Under close supervision, warfarin can be used in combination with aspirin.

Heparin is the classic intravenous anticoagulant used in hospitals. Newer agents called low molecular weight heparins have been developed (enoxaparin, dalteparin) that are purer forms of heparin. They work better for some people. For instance, enoxaparin has proven to be superior to heparin for people with unstable angina and heart attack. Fondaparinux (*Arixtra*) is a new synthetic blood thinner that has shown promise.

In rare cases, some people may be allergic to all heparin-based drugs. If you're one of these individuals, your cardiologist will prescribe an alternate medication when you're hospitalized.

Commonly prescribed oral anticoagulant: warfarin (*Coumadin*)

Precautions When Taking Blood-Thinning Medications

If you're taking any type of blood-thinning medication:

- Take the medication exactly as your doctor instructs.
- Ask your doctor before taking other medications or supplements, even vitamins or over-the-counter medications.
- Ask for any interactions with foods (vitamin K in broccoli and spinach).
- Be sure to have blood tests regularly so your doctor can monitor how well your medications are working.
- Tell your doctor about these (and any other medications you're taking) before you have surgery.
- Watch for warning signs and let your doctor know right away if you have:
  - pink or red urine
  - red, black, or dark brown stools
  - heavy menstrual bleeding (more than normal)
  - bleeding gums

Report these conditions to your physician:

- intense headache or stomach pain that doesn't go away
- weakness, dizziness, fainting, or a general feeling of being unwell
- bruises or blood blisters
- pregnancy
- an accident of any kind (which could cause bleeding)

Thrombolytics

These clot-busting drugs are used to dissolve blood clots during a heart attack. They work by increasing the blood level and action of an enzyme (*plasmin*) that breaks up blood clots. While thrombolytics can't prevent a heart attack, they can help you survive one. To be effective, thrombolytics must be administered within the first few hours of a heart attack. They're most effective if they're given within the first hour; the hospitals should administer this medication within thirty minutes of a patient's arrival at a hospital emergency room.

The major risk with thrombolytics is bleeding, especially bleeding into the brain. This is relatively rare (up to 1.5 percent of cases) and occurs more frequently in women over the age of seventy.

Commonly prescribed thrombolytics: tissue plasminogen activator or tPA (*Activase*), reteplase or rPA (*Retavase*), tenecteplase (*TNK*), and streptokinase (*Kabikinase, Streptase*). Note: angioplasty and stenting have replaced thrombolytics as the treatment of choice for heart attacks.

Cholesterol-Lowering Medications

If you have CHD, one of your treatment goals will be to reduce your LDL cholesterol to 100 mg/dL or less (ideally, less than 70 mg/dL). In addition to lifestyle changes, your doctor may prescribe cholesterol-lowering medications. All cholesterol-lowering medications are used with dietary therapy and need to be taken for at least a few years, sometimes for life.

A variety of drugs are available for lowering cholesterol. Common types include *statins, ezetimibe, fibrates, resins, nicotinic acid*, and omega-3 fish oil. Your doctor may prescribe a combination of drugs, especially if a single cholesterol-lowering medication doesn't improve your cholesterol levels.

Statins

Statins are fast becoming the drugs of choice for reducing cholesterol. Statins enhance the body's ability to rid itself of cholesterol. They work directly on the liver to block a substance your body needs to manufacture cholesterol. The result is that cholesterol in the liver becomes depleted and cholesterol is removed from the circulating blood.

Statins are especially effective in reducing LDL cholesterol. Some studies indicate that statins can reduce LDL cholesterol by 30 to 40 percent, usually enough to bring cholesterol levels within safe limits. Statins may also help the body reabsorb cholesterol from plaques, slowly reversing atherosclerosis. Statins have been proven to reduce the risk of a second heart attack and the risk of death from CHD.

Statins are easy to take, have few drug interactions, and have few short-term side effects. Your doctor should monitor your liver function and test for muscle inflammation to ensure the drugs are not causing any problems. A rare side effect is a serious muscle breakdown called *rhabdomyolysis*, which tends to occur when taking both a statin and a fibrate for high triglycerides. Warning signs of muscle damage would include: dark urine and muscle aches, weakness, fever, nausea, and vomiting. At the first sign of these problems, stop taking the medication immediately and contact your doctor. If caught early, problems from this uncommon side effect can be quickly and effectively treated.

Statins also should not be used if you're pregnant or if you have chronic liver disease. In a few cases, people are allergic to statins and need to choose other cholesterol-lowering drugs.

Because the body makes more cholesterol at night, statins are usually taken two hours after dinner or at bedtime. The drugs take four to six weeks to be effective. Avoid drinking grapefruit juice if you're taking certain statins since it can interfere with your body's ability to clear some of these drugs from the liver.

Commonly prescribed statins: atorvastatin (*Lipitor*), fluvastatin (*Lescol*), lovastatin (*Mevacor*), pravastatin (*Pravachol*), rosuvastatin (*Crestor*), and simvastatin (*Zocor*)

Ezetimibe (Zetia)

Unlike statins, which work mainly on the liver to decrease the production of cholesterol, *ezetimibe* works in the digestive tract. It targets the cholesterol that comes from food and reduces the amount absorbed by the body. When a healthful diet and exercise do not lower your cholesterol enough, ezetimibe may be recommended to complement these efforts. Ezetimibe may be prescribed alone or your doctor may recommend taking ezetimibe in addition to a statin. Studies have shown that LDL cholesterol is lowered by an average of thirty points, or 18 percent, when ezetimibe is taken in conjunction with diet and exercise. One clinical study showed that people already taking statins who added ezetimibe saw their LDL cholesterol drop by an average of an additional 25 percent (about thirty-six points).

Although ezetimibe reduces the amount of cholesterol that's absorbed from food, it doesn't give you license to throw your diet

---

If your doctor prescribes cholesterol-lowering medication, you will also need to:

- Follow a cholesterol-lowering diet
- Be physically active (as recommended by your doctor)
- Lose excess weight if you're overweight
- Stop smoking
- Control your high blood pressure and diabetes

---

out the window and indulge in foods that are high in saturated fat and cholesterol. Likewise, the medication won't help you lose weight.

Ezetimibe is generally well tolerated with few side effects, including stomach pain and feeling tired. However, experiencing unexplained weakness or muscle pain could be a sign of a rare but serious side effect and should be reported to your doctor. In some cases, your doctor may do blood tests to check the health of your liver prior to prescribing ezetimibe; he or she may also check your liver periodically as you continue to take the medication. If you've ever had liver disease, you may not be a candidate for ezetimibe. A combination pill is available in the form of ezetimibe and simvastatin called *Vytorin*.

Fibrates

These drugs are mainly triglyceride-lowering medications. Fibrates reduce the production of triglycerides and remove them from circulation. They do this by stimulating the *lipoprotein lipase*, an enzyme that breaks down lipids in lipoproteins. Studies have shown that fibrates can reduce triglycerides by 20 to 50 percent and increase "good" HDL cholesterol by 10 to 15 percent. Fibrates also mildly reduce LDL cholesterol levels, but the drugs haven't been approved for this purpose.

Most people have few side effects with fibrates, although some experience gastrointestinal problems such as gas or bloating. The drugs also increase the likelihood of developing cholesterol gallstones. Fibrates can also magnify the effect of blood-thinning medications.

Commonly prescribed fibrates: fenofibrate (*Tricor, Triglide*) and gemfibrozil (*Lopid*)

Resins

Used for cholesterol lowering for at least twenty years, resins (also called bile acid sequestrants) cause the intestines to absorb less cholesterol from the digestive tract. The body normally makes bile acids from cholesterol and passes them from the liver into the intestines. Some acids, however, return to the bloodstream through the intestine wall. Bile acid–binding drugs like resins don't allow the bile acids to return to the bloodstream. They also force more of the cholesterol in the liver to make bile acids, resulting in less cholesterol to reach the bloodstream. Over time, this process reduces blood cholesterol. Studies have shown that resins lower LDL cholesterol by 10 to 20 percent. For people with CHD, these drugs are sometimes combined with statins to increase their effectiveness. This combination can often reduce LDL cholesterol by as much as 40 percent.

Resins are available in tablet and powder forms. The powders must be mixed with water or fruit juice and usually are taken one to two times a day with meals. Drinking large amounts of water and other liquids can help prevent gastrointestinal problems such as gas, nausea, bloating, and constipation.

Commonly prescribed resins: cholestyramine (*Questran*), colestipol (*Colestid*), and colesevelam (*WelChol*)

Nicotinic Acid

Niacin is a water-soluble B vitamin. In the form of *nicotinic acid*, in large doses it can lower triglycerides and "bad" LDL cholesterol; it can also change the LDL particles to a larger, less dangerous size. Niacin can also increase "good" HDL cholesterol. (Nicotinic acid shouldn't be confused with *nicotinamide*, another form of niacin which doesn't lower cholesterol.)

Nicotinic acid is available as an immediate-release drug (*Niacor*) and in a timed-released and extended-release form (*Niaspan*). In the past, most heart experts recommended the immediate-release type. Now, the longer-acting Niaspan is more often prescribed. Even though it's more expensive, Niaspan has the convenience of once-a-day dosing and fewer side effects. Talk with your doctor about which drug is best for you.

Nicotinic acid is widely available without a prescription. However, it should not be used for cholesterol lowering without a doctor's supervision due to potential side effects. These side effects include flushing, which can be quite uncomfortable. If you experience flushing, patches of your skin will turn red and you'll feel burning sensations. Flushing can be lessened by taking an aspirin one hour before taking the nicotinic acid. Other side effects include itching and stomach upset.

Taking nicotinic acid with high blood pressure medicines can increase the effects of the blood pressure medication. If you're using this drug combination, it's important that your blood pressure be carefully monitored. Nicotinic acid can also cause liver problems, gout, and an increase in blood sugar levels. If you have diabetes, gout, or stomach ulcers, your doctor may choose a different cholesterol-lowering medication.

Commonly prescribed nicotinic acid: Niacor, Niaspan

Combination statin and niacin: Advicor (lovastatin and extended-release niacin)

Nonmedication Treatment for Lowering Cholesterol

In this chapter we have discussed medications that are effective in lowering "bad" cholesterol levels. However, when diet, exercise, and medications don't succeed in lowering cholesterol, a medical procedure, *LDL apheresis*, is another treatment option. Also called *cholesterol apheresis*, this minimally invasive procedure is a filtering process; it involves drawing the blood from a vein and passing it through a machine that separates it from the plasma. While the blood is returned to the body through a different vein, the plasma passes through another part of the machine where the bad cholesterol is physically removed. As the treated plasma is returned to the body, "bad" LDL levels are dramatically reduced, helping to prevent heart attacks and stroke.

LDL apheresis is designed primarily for patients with CHD and an LDL level of above 200 mg/dL or for those who don't have CHD but who have LDL levels of 300 mg/dL or higher.

Although this procedure is effective, it is time-consuming. Each treatment takes approximately two to four hours and must be repeated every two to three weeks. Other than possibly being asked to refrain from taking any ACE inhibitors, which are discussed below, there are no preparations required before treatment. However, finding a treatment center can be difficult—there are only about twenty centers throughout the nation offering LDL apheresis.

Medications to Lower Blood Pressure

ACE Inhibitors

ACE (angiotensin converting enzyme) inhibitors are a class of drugs that block the formation of angiotensin, a potent chemical that causes tiny arteries to constrict. They are effective in lowering high blood pressure. They help heal the heart muscle after a heart attack and lower the death rate of people with weakened hearts. For people with diabetes, they protect kidney function.

ACE drugs, like other medications, have side effects. The most serious one is kidney failure in people who have narrowing of both kidney arteries, a condition detectable by ultrasound. The most common side effect of ACE drugs is a dry, hacking cough, which is reversible. These drugs can also cause some people to develop high levels of potassium in the blood. If you take an ACE inhibitor, your doctor will want to monitor your potassium blood levels and kidney function regularly.

ACE inhibitors should not be used during pregnancy. Low blood pressure, severe kidney failure, excess potassium, and even death in the newborn can occur. If you're pregnant or think you might be pregnant, inform your doctor immediately.

Commonly prescribed ACEs: benazepril (*Lotensin*), captopril (*Capoten*), fosinopril (*Monopril*), enalapril (*Vasotec*), lisinopril (*Prinivil, Zestril*), ramipril (*Altace*), quinapril (*Accupril*), and trandolapril (*Mavik*)

ARBs

Angiotensin receptor blockers (ARBs) directly block the effects of angiotensin, the chemical that causes tiny arteries to constrict. They are effective in lowering blood pressure and, for diabetics, protecting kidney function. ARBs are an alternative medication for people with heart attack or heart failure who cannot use ACEs. A dry cough isn't as big a problem with ARBs as it is with ACEs but still can occur in 3 to 5 percent of people. ARBs can cause birth defects and shouldn't be taken during pregnancy. Inform your doctor immediately if you're pregnant or think you might be pregnant.

Commonly prescribed ARBs: candesartan (*Atacand*), irbesartan (*Avapro*), losartan (*Cozaar, Hyzaar*), olmesartan (*Benicar*), telmisartan (*Micardis*), and valsartan (*Diovan*)

Diuretics

Commonly called "water pills," these drugs flush excess water and sodium (salt) from the body by increasing urination. This reduces the amount of fluid and sodium in the blood, lowering blood pressure.

Diuretics include: hydrochlorthiazide (*HCTZ, Hydodiuril*), chlorthalidone (*Hygroton*), indapamide (*Lozol*), furosemide (*Lasix*), torsemide (*Demedex*), bumetanide (*Bumex*), and metolazone (*Zaroxolyn*)

Beta-Blockers

Beta-blockers reduce blood pressure by decreasing heart rate, reducing the strength of the heart's contractions, and relaxing blood vessel walls. For people who have CHD and high blood pressure, a combination of beta-blockers and ACE inhibitors is the preferred treatment. See anti-anginal medications earlier in this chapter for more information on beta-blockers.

Calcium Channel Blockers

These drugs relax the blood vessels and reduce blood pressure by preventing calcium from entering the muscle cells of the heart. See anti-anginal medications earlier in this chapter for more information on calcium channel blockers.

Alpha-Blockers

These drugs lower blood pressure by blocking the stimulation of specialized nerves. Alpha-blockers are often used to treat urinary frequency caused by an enlarged prostate gland.

Commonly prescribed alpha-blockers: doxazosin mesylate (*Cardura*), prazosin hydrochloride (*Minipress*), and terazosin hydrochloride (*Hytrin*)

Nerve Inhibitors

The sympathetic nerves extend from the brain to all parts of the body, including the arteries and their tiny branches. Nerve-inhibiting drugs reduce blood pressure by affecting control centers in the brain that keep these nerves from narrowing (constricting) blood vessels. They can be very effective, but their use is limited because they cause fatigue and dry mouth.

Commonly prescribed nerve inhibitor: clonidine (*Catapres*)

Vasodilators

These medications reduce blood pressure by causing the muscle in the walls of the blood vessels, especially the tiny arterioles, to widen or relax. Because they may also cause the body to retain salt and water and speed heart rate, they're often prescribed in combination with diuretics and beta-blockers.

Commonly prescribed vasodilators: hydralazine hydrochloride (*Apresoline*) and minoxidil (*Loniten*)

Getting the Most Benefit from Your Medications

Regardless of the type of medication your doctor prescribes, follow these tips to make taking your medications easier, safer, and more effective.

- Always talk with your doctor and/or pharmacist before taking over-the-counter medications, vitamins and minerals, or herbal supplements. Some medications can dangerously interact or become less effective when used with other substances.

- Use one pharmacy for all your medications, preferably one that uses computerized drug tracking, to avoid possible dangerous drug interactions.
- Understand how and why you're taking different medications. If you're uncertain, talk with your doctor and/or pharmacist.
- Read labels and any written information that comes with the medicine before taking it. Be sure to read the warnings.
- Ask your doctor or pharmacist before crushing, splitting, or chewing any medication. Some types of medication should only be taken whole.
- If you have side effects or develop new symptoms, talk with your doctor right away. Sometimes the doctor can adjust your medication or have you take it at a different time or in a different way to minimize side effects.
- Take only as much medication as prescribed.
- Don't skip doses or stop taking your medication without your doctor's permission, even if you're feeling better. Some medications need to be tapered off slowly to avoid problems.
- Keep all appointments for tests that monitor your medications. Some drugs have potentially harmful effects and need to be carefully monitored.
- Toss out any medication that has passed its expiration date. Some outdated medications lose their potency; others may become dangerous as they break down over time.

- Never share your medications or take anyone else's medications.
- Organize your medications so that they're easy to take, especially if you take a number of drugs or take them at different times. Pharmacies carry medication reminder devices such as containers that beep, special caps that count how often a prescription bottle has been opened, and computerized drug organizer-dispensers. Putting your medications where you'll see them, keeping them in sectioned containers, taking them at specific times of the day (e.g., mealtimes), and even checking off a calendar as you take them can help keep you on track.
- Keep a current list of all your medications, including the names, dosages, and when and how you take them. Review this list with your doctor and your pharmacist to ensure you aren't taking medications that may dangerously interact. Let your doctor know about any medications that have caused you problems in the past such as rashes, dizziness, indigestion, or poor appetite.
- Store your medicines in a cool, dry place (unless otherwise directed) in their original containers. Because bathrooms tend to be hot and moist, they are not good storage places for drugs. Keep all medicines away from children.
- If you are pregnant or considering becoming pregnant, consult your doctor about all drugs you are taking.

8 Angioplasty, Stents, and Bypass Surgery

Many people are able to control coronary heart disease with healthful lifestyle changes and medications. However, if the blockages in your coronary arteries are severe or if you continue to have frequent or disabling chest discomfort (angina) despite the use of medication, you may need other treatments to improve the blood supply to your heart. Having more blood get to your heart should help reduce or eliminate angina, reduce fatigue, and possibly decrease your need for medication. These additional therapies can improve the quality and the length of your life.

The first of these medical treatments is a procedure called *coronary balloon angioplasty*, more commonly known as *percutaneous coronary intervention (PCI)*. The second is *bypass surgery*, a more extensive procedure, which is technically known as *coronary artery bypass graft surgery (CABG)*. While anti-anginal medications generally work by decreasing the heart's need for oxygen and nutrients, balloon angioplasty and bypass surgery are designed to increase the supply.

Coronary Angioplasty and Stents

Coronary balloon angioplasty is a minimally invasive surgical procedure used to restore blood flow through an artery that has become blocked by plaque buildup. Angioplasty is used to relieve chest pain caused by a reduction in blood flow to the heart and to minimize damage to the heart muscle as the result of an evolving (in progress) heart attack. During the procedure, a tiny balloon is used to widen the artery without the need to surgically open the chest. Once the blockage is partially cleared, a stent, which is a tiny mesh tube, is inserted to keep the artery open. Stents are used in more than 90 percent of angioplasty procedures.

However, when stents were first introduced in the 1990s, it was soon discovered that scar tissue developed inside the stents of 20 to 35 percent of patients; this scar tissue buildup, called *restenosis* (renarrowing), created new blockages at the treatment site.

In an effort to eliminate restenosis, medical researchers developed *drug-eluting* or *drug-coated stents (DES)*, which reduce the buildup of scar tissue and increase the likelihood that arteries will remain open. Approved by the Food and Drug Administration in 2003, these are the most popular stents used today. They have a renarrowing rate of less than 5 to 10 percent in most patients, compared to the 20 to 35 percent in patients with conventional, nonmedicated stents, also known as *bare metal stents* or *BMS*. Reducing the risk of renarrowing means fewer patients require a return visit to the catheterization lab, and fewer ultimately need bypass surgery.

Are Drug-Coated Stents Safe?

In 2006, questions arose about the safety of drug-coated stents. Although the stents helped prevent arteries from renarrowing, research showed that more than a year after receiving the medicated stents, a small number of patients, approximately one in 500, faced a greater risk of forming blood clots and having potentially fatal heart attacks. Originally, patients with newly placed stents were prescribed aspirin to be taken indefinitely and the anti-clotting drug *clopidgrel* or *Plavix* for up to 12 months. However, with the information about the rare but real increased risk of heart attack, a physician may recommend that a patient continue taking aspirin indefinitely and Plavix for a more prolonged period of time. It is important that you and your cardiologist discuss the risks of a stented artery renarrowing versus the risk of blood clots. If non-cardiac surgery is planned or if the patient cannot reliably take long-term Plavix, a bare metal stent may be a better option.

Other Improvements in Stent Technology

In addition to the drug-coated stents, other advancements have been made in angioplasty and the tools used to perform it. The *interventional cardiologist*, a doctor who specializes in performing angioplasty and other catheter-based surgical interventions, now has tools adapted to treat specific types of narrowing arteries.

For instance, to treat calcified plaque the cardiologist uses a diamond-coated burr that spins at 180,000 revolutions per minute in a technique called *rotational atherectomy*. The burr breaks through the plaque and creates a smooth artery channel. Once the plaque is shattered into tiny bits, the body clears the plaque debris through its own disposal system in the liver, spleen, and bone marrow. In experienced hands, rotational atherectomy has made angioplasty safer for treating complex blockages. Rotational atherectomy is commonly followed by the insertion of a stent to decrease renarrowing.

Another advancement, *intravascular ultrasound (IVUS)*, also known as *intravascular echocardiography*, combines cardiac catheterization and echocardiography to see directly inside the coronary arteries. This advanced technique allows doctors to thread a tiny ultrasound "camera" into the coronary arteries and uses sound waves to produce a cross-sectional image of the inside walls of the arteries. With this view, doctors can discern plaque levels, measure the artery size more precisely, and better determine which size and type of stent to use for an angioplasty procedure. Once the stent is in place, they can also verify that the stent has been placed properly.

Another improvement in technology is the *pressure wire*, which is inserted via a catheter. This diagnostic tool is used in the catheter lab to help determine whether a narrowing is severe enough to be treated with angioplasty. The wire has a sensor that measures the pressure in the artery on both sides of the narrowing. The differences in the pressures can reveal the significance of the blockage.

Finally, different types of protection devices such as balloons with *suction devices*, *mini-umbrellas*, and *filters on wires* help in the treatment of prior bypass grafts that have developed plaque buildup or blood clots. These devices minimize debris from plaque going downstream and blocking the small arteries of the heart, which can cause heart attacks.

Undergoing an Angioplasty-Stenting Procedure

Angioplasty and stenting are typically performed in a catheterization suite or "cath" lab in a hospital. Patients are given local anesthesia and sedation with a relaxant medication similar to Valium. The procedure takes thirty minutes to two hours, depending on

Stent Insertion

The top illustration shows the collapsed stent being guided into the artery. In the middle illustration, the stent is being expanded by a balloon. The bottom illustration shows the stent in place; the balloon has been withdrawn.

the extent of blockages. In most cases, it requires only an over-night hospital stay.

The Procedure

During the angioplasty-stenting procedure, your heart rate and rhythm will be monitored. After numbing the area with a local anesthetic, your cardiologist will make a small incision in your leg or your groin (less often in your arm). Then he or she will insert a long, narrow, hollow tube, called a guide catheter, through the artery. Guided by X-ray images on a television monitor, the doctor will move the catheter through the artery to the blockage. During this time, you may feel some discomfort—chest heaviness, discomfort in the arm, and/or shortness of breath; however, most people report the procedure isn't painful. At this point, the doctor will inject a small amount of X-ray dye or "contrast." This will enable the cardiologist to see the exact location of the blockage.

Once the guiding catheter is in the right place, a second, smaller catheter equipped with a deflated balloon which tracks over a very thin wire (14/1000 of an inch) is inserted into the guide catheter. After the wire is threaded across the narrowing, the deflated balloon is moved into the blockage area. The doctor inflates the balloon for fifteen to sixty seconds on average to widen the artery and then deflates it. The doctor may repeat the inflation-deflation several times. During this part of the procedure, you may feel chest pain or pressure, which is similar to the discomfort you may have experienced prior to the procedure. That's because while the balloon is inflated, blood flow through the artery is temporarily blocked. Let the doctor know if you feel pain. In most cases, the pain goes away once the balloon is deflated.

Next, the cardiologist will usually insert a stent, the fine wire-mesh tube for propping open the artery. The stent is mounted on a balloon angioplasty catheter in a collapsed state, moved to the blockage area where the balloon is inflated, and inserted. The balloon is then deflated and removed, leaving the expanded stent in place. Stents are designed to stay in the artery permanently. Some patients may require more than one stent in an artery; or they may need stents in more than one artery, depending on the number and locations of the narrowing.

Once the balloon catheter is removed, pictures (angiograms) are taken to see how well blood is flowing through the affected artery. In some cases, results are confirmed with an intravascular ultrasound (IVUS), which produces a picture from inside the arteries. If blood is flowing well, the guide catheter will be removed. About two to four hours later, when the blood thinners you've been given have been neutralized by the body, the sheath or plastic tube through which the catheter was inserted will be removed. Some physicians use a plug or stitch at the time of the procedure to seal the access site.

The Recovery

The medical team will watch your recovery carefully for twelve to twenty-four hours. Be sure to let the nurses or doctor know if you feel any pain or discomfort following your angioplasty procedure.

Your doctor will order oral, and when indicated, intravenous blood-thinning medication to prevent clot formation. You may also be given nitroglycerine to relax the coronary arteries, and calcium antagonists to protect the arteries from spasm.

You'll need to return to your doctor within a couple of weeks and then within six months to evaluate how well the procedure is keeping the artery open. The follow-up, which involves a checkup, ECG, and/or nuclear stress tests, can be done in your doctor's office. These procedures are noninvasive and painless. If a stress test indicates it's safe, your doctor may recommend a *cardiac rehabilitation program*—a structured plan of education, exercise, and other lifestyle changes to reduce your cardiac risk factors.

How Effective is Angioplasty?

More than 500,000 angioplasty/stent procedures are performed in the United States every year. Worldwide, it's estimated that more than one million are performed annually. For many people, the procedure relieves angina better than medication alone. With the availability and use of stents, success rates for treating arteries that are not totally blocked exceed 95 percent. The success of treating total blockages with angioplasty depends largely on how long the artery has been totally blocked. If the artery has been completely blocked for less than three months, the angioplasty success rate is above 80 percent. It drops to less than 50 percent if the artery has been completely blocked for more than three months.

Angioplasty/stenting is easier for the patient and less invasive than coronary artery bypass graft surgery (CABG). It doesn't involve general anesthesia, it's less expensive, hospital stays are shorter, and recovery time is faster. Major complications are unusual. If the procedure needs to be repeated, the risks are no higher than the initial procedure, whereas a repeat bypass operation is riskier than the first. This risk, however, depends on the distribution of the blockage(s).

At left, the photo shows narrowing in the left descending artery (LAD). The right illustration shows the same artery after placement of a stent.

How Safe is Angioplasy?

Overall, the angioplasty procedure is relatively safe. Less than 1 percent of patients who undergo angioplasty need emergency bypass surgery during the procedure. The risk of death from angioplasty is less than 1 percent. The risk of having a minor heart attack during the procedure is 2 to 6 percent, a major heart attack less than 1 percent. The incidence of heart attack, stroke, and death following angioplasty is higher for women than for men. This may be because women who undergo the procedure tend to be older and have a higher incidence of high blood pressure, diabetes, high blood cholesterol, and other health problems than men who undergo the procedure.

In addition to the rare risks of heart attack, stroke, and death, other complications may occur. These complications are usually treatable. They include:

- injury or puncture of the artery during insertion of the catheter
- increased risk of clot formation inside the artery
- blockages made worse if the angioplasty causes scar tissue to form, creating greater blockage

Your physician must advise you of the risk of not treating your CHD blockages weighed against the risk of complications.

Who Is a Candidate for Angioplasty?

Previously, angioplasty was performed only on people who had one severely blocked artery. Now, due to advances in the procedure, doctors are using angioplasty even on people with severe and multiple blockages. Studies show that the procedure provides more complete relief than medication alone for people with angina. Depending on where the blockages are located, angioplasty is equivalent to bypass surgery in providing relief from angina, in risk of heart attack, and in long-term survival rates. The exceptions are patients with narrowing of the main artery or *left main coronary artery* and diabetics who have significant blockages in one of the major coronary arteries (*left anterior descending artery* or *LAD*). Studies are ongoing with these groups of patients

Whether angioplasty or the more invasive coronary bypass surgery is right for you is a decision you and your doctor will have to make together, depending on:

- the location of your blockages
- how many blockages you have
- how extensive the blockages are
- your age

- your overall health
- how well your heart is functioning
- how hardened (calcified) your plaques are
- whether you have a valve problem that would benefit from surgery

You may *not* be a candidate for angioplasty if:

- your heart disease is too advanced
- the plaque is located in an area inaccessible by catheter (too far or in a curve in the artery)
- the plaque is severely calcified (In skilled hands, rotational atherectomy is usually successful.)
- the plaque is in the main left coronary artery
- blockage is complete in one or more coronary arteries (especially if the artery has been blocked for a long time)

If you're not a candidate for angioplasty, coronary bypass surgery may be more appropriate for you.

Coronary Artery Bypass Graft Surgery (CABG)

Although angioplasty is an effective treatment for many, it's not always the best treatment for everyone. Some individuals may do better with *coronary bypass*, also known as coronary artery bypass graft surgery (CABG, pronounced "cabbage"). It is a major surgical procedure, that increases blood supply to the heart. The bypass procedure involves taking a piece of a blood vessel, usually from the chest and/or leg, and stitching it onto the blocked artery, replenishing blood supply. Think of it as a detour, which goes around the problem site—the blockage. In many cases, more than one artery is blocked, requiring multiple bypasses.

Bypass surgery may be an option for blockages that can't be adequately treated with angioplasty. This might include people who have arteries that are chronically totally blocked, narrowing in all the coronary arteries, and/or narrowing in the left main coronary artery. Also, people who are diabetic and have narrowings in the artery that supplies the front of the heart (left anterior descending artery or LAD) have better results with bypass surgery, especially if the narrowings involve long segments of clogged arteries.

Who Is a Candidate for Bypass Surgery?

In general, bypass surgery is used when coronary blockages are severe and widespread, especially if three arteries are blocked or the blockages occur at critical locations in the heart's circulatory system. Because bypass is a major operation, your doctor will recommend it only after careful consideration. In addition to assessing the location and extent of your blockages, your doctor will consider the overall health of your heart, your age, and other non-heart health problems you may have.

If you have a choice of undergoing angioplasty or bypass surgery, ask your doctor about the risks and benefits of each. Consider getting a second or even a third opinion before making your decision.

You may be a candidate for bypass surgery if:

- Your angina is debilitating and interferes with normal functions of daily life.
- Two or all three main coronary arteries are narrowed 75 percent or more. (Some people with CHD in only one vessel may also benefit.)

- The left main coronary artery is 70 percent or more narrowed (50 percent in some cases).
- You have poor function of the left ventricle, the heart's main pumping station, which may improve with a renewed blood supply.
- You have a very abnormal exercise or nuclear test despite the absence of symptoms.
- You're not a good candidate for angioplasty/stenting.
- You've already undergone a catheter treatment that's been unsuccessful.
- Bypasses from a previous operation have closed.

Before Surgery

Once you're admitted to the hospital, you'll be given blood and urine tests, a chest X-ray, ECG, and other tests. Unless you've already had angiograms taken, a diagnostic cardiac catheterization or angiography will be performed. The images will serve as a road map that enables your surgeon to know where to place the bypasses. The night before your surgery, you'll shower with a special soap to decrease the risk of infection.

You'll probably take your regular medications, but you should ask your doctor first. Your doctor will likely have you not take aspirin or other blood-thinning medications to avoid the risk of bleeding during and immediately following the surgery. (Urgent bypass surgeries are frequently done while the patient is taking these medications and blood transfusions are more often required.) A nurse will prepare you for surgery by shaving your chest and legs. About an hour before surgery, you'll be given a sedative to help you relax. Once you're in the operating room, the anesthesiologist will give you a general anesthetic to put you to sleep.

Bypass Grafts

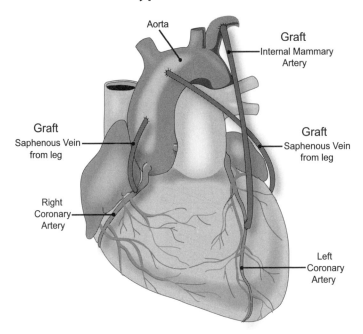

Bypass grafts are shown here. Using magnification, surgeons use hair-fine sutures to attach the grafts.

He or she will insert a special intravenous line to help monitor your blood pressure and the pressure inside your lungs during the operation.

The Bypass Procedure

The procedure takes two to five hours, depending on the number of bypasses and the complexity of the surgery. To begin the operation, your surgeon will expose your heart by making an incision through the middle of the chest and through the breast-bone. Once the heart is exposed, you may be put on the *heart-*

lung bypass, or *pump oxygenator*. Specialized health professionals called *perfusionists* operate this machine. The heart-lung machine oxygenates the blood like the lungs would. Then it pumps the blood into the aorta downstream from the heart, where it flows to all the organs. While you're on the heart-lung bypass, your heart is stopped and blood doesn't flow to it (what surgeons call a "bloodless field"). This allows the surgeon to work precisely on the heart while it's not moving. To ensure the heart isn't damaged during this time, the heart is cooled and chemicals are added to reduce its need for oxygen.

The bypass arteries and/or veins are delicately sewn into place. The average is three or four bypasses. Once the grafts are in place, the heart is rewarmed. The surgeon uses electric shock to restart the heart and then closes the incisions.

Harvesting Blood Vessels for Bypass

Many people are concerned about the blood vessels used in bypass. Won't you miss them? Won't the area from which they're taken suffer? The answer to both questions is generally no. The arteries or veins used in bypass aren't essential. Removing, or "harvesting," them doesn't significantly impact the blood flow from where they're taken. The *internal mammary artery (IMA)* (also called the *internal thoracic artery*), located on the inside chest wall, is used in more than 90 percent of bypass procedures. We have two mammary arteries: one on the left and one on the right side of the chest. (The right mammary artery is used less often in bypass.) The mammary arteries tend to stay open longer than other blood vessels that can be used. When a mammary artery is used, an additional incision is not required, and the surgeon usually doesn't have to entirely remove it. Instead, he or she reconnects the downstream part of the mammary artery to the coronary artery, bypassing the blockage.

Most bypasses use some of the superficial (saphenous) vein that runs down the inside of the leg. Sometimes veins are taken from both legs. A specially trained *physician assistant (PA)* or an assisting surgeon will make another incision on the inside of one or both legs to remove the vein. New endoscopic minimally invasive techniques are now used, minimizing the incision length to a few inches and lowering the risk of complications. Once the vein is removed, one end of it is connected to the aorta and the other to the coronary artery downstream from the blockage. Less commonly, veins may be taken from the backs of the legs or arms. Sometimes the artery that supplies blood to the hand (the radial artery) is used if the other hand artery (the ulnar artery) can provide an adequate supply of blood to the hand. If needed, an artery in the abdomen can be redirected and used as a bypass graft.

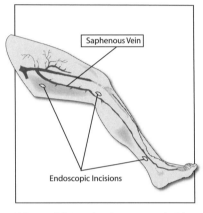

Saphenous Vein

Endoscopic Incisions

When additional veins are needed for bypass surgery, the saphenous vein, which runs down the inside of the leg, is often used.

Recovery from Bypass Surgery

After surgery, you'll be taken to a cardiac surgery recovery area or intensive care unit for twenty-four to thirty-six hours. Small tubes in your chest and arms will remain in place for twenty-four hours. These tubes allow the doctors to check for internal bleeding, give drugs and fluids, withdraw blood samples, drain off fluid, and continuously monitor your blood pressure. Small patches (electrodes) on your chest let the staff monitor your heart's rate and rhythm with the ECG. A breathing tube (*endotracheal tube*) that goes through your mouth into your windpipe will help you breathe. It's usually removed within the first twenty-four hours.

After the first twenty-four hours following surgery, recovery is usually fairly quick. You should be alert and able to eat and walk. If you've had one or more veins removed from your legs, you may need to wear elastic support stockings to help circulation and reduce swelling. About 20 percent of people who undergo bypass surgery require a blood transfusion following surgery. Thirty to forty percent develop erratic heart rhythm problems (atrial fibrillation) that require special care, but these are easily treated in most cases. A few patients develop infection at the wound site. Barring these complications, you should be able to leave the hospital in four to six days.

You'll need to see your doctor in a week or so to have any external stitches or staples removed from your chest. If you have leg stitches, they'll need to stay in a few days longer. Most people have absorbable stitches that are placed under the skin and disappear on their own. The incision is closed on the outside with a special tape.

Your surgical wounds should heal within six weeks or so. If you have a sedentary job, you'll likely be able to return to work in about four weeks. If you have a physically demanding occupation, you may need to wait six weeks or longer. Your doctor will usually recommend a monitored exercise program. You may participate in the program while you are working in a light job. However, if you have a job requiring heavy physical labor, you'll probably need to complete the monitored exercise program before returning to work.

During recovery, it's important to avoid heavy lifting and take time to build up your endurance. You can't drive for six weeks. At first you'll likely feel weak and tired. That's understandable, considering that a week in bed shrinks muscle strength by 15 percent. It also takes a lot of energy for your body to heal itself. Walking is a great way to regain your strength and energy. You'll want to keep an eye out for warning signs of infection, fluid retention, or problems with your bypasses, including:

- redness or drainage at the incision site
- fever
- chills
- increasing fatigue
- weight gain over five pounds in a few days
- changes in heart rate or rhythms (palpitations or skipped beats)
- swollen ankles (Often the leg from which the vein was taken swells more, making the legs feel unequal.)

Is Coronary Bypass Surgery Safe?

Coronary artery bypass is major surgery and carries risks. The biggest risk, of course, is dying. The overall risk of dying from bypass surgery is 1 to 2 percent. For women, it's slightly higher. It still means that 98 to 99 percent of people who undergo bypass surgery will survive. If you must undergo the surgery during an emergency situation such as a heart attack, your risk of dying increases to 5 to 8 percent. Fortunately, emergency surgery is less common than it was prior to the availability of stents. The risks are also higher for people who are older or who have extensive scarring from previous heart attacks.

Coronary artery bypass substantially improves symptoms in 90 percent of those who undergo the operation. However, sometimes narrowings develop in the bypasses themselves. Ten years after surgery, one-third of venous bypasses are closed, one-third are narrowed, and one-third remain wide open. The results with mammary artery bypasses are better—a full 96 percent remain open after ten years. On average, the five-year survival rate for men who have undergone bypass is 90 to 94 percent. For women, the five-year survival rate is 87 to 91 percent. (A five-year survival rate means that an individual will be alive *at least* five years later.)

Newer Bypass Techniques

As mentioned earlier in this chapter, coronary bypass surgery has traditionally required the use of a heart-lung machine to keep blood flowing and allow the surgeon to stop your heart so that the bypasses can be precisely connected.

Recently, less invasive forms of bypass surgery are being performed. One procedure, called *minimally invasive direct coronary artery bypass* or *MIDCAB*, has become popular because it can be performed on a beating heart, eliminating the need to place the patient on the heart-lung machine. Since the patient's is not "on" the heart-lung machine, the procedure is said to be "off pump."

For the MIDCAB, a smaller incision is made in the chest directly over the artery or arteries to be bypassed. The surgeon detaches an artery, usually from inside the chest, and reattaches it to the clogged artery beyond the blockage. MIDCAB is generally used when only one or two arteries need to be bypassed. Patients undergoing this type of surgery usually have shorter hospital stays.

A variation of MIDCAB, a procedure called *off-pump coronary artery bypass (OPCAB)*, is used more often. Here, the cardiac surgeon does not enter the chest cavity through small holes; instead, he/she makes a chest incision like that used in a standard bypass operation; but the heart-lung machine isn't used, making it an "off pump" procedure. The surgeon works on the heart while it's beating, often attaching several bypasses. Both these off-pump procedures require that the operating room be ready to place a patient on the heart-lung machine if complications should occur.

These newer procedures are being carefully evaluated. A recent major comparison of both techniques—the use of the heart-lung machine and off pump—showed the success of the bypasses were similar. However, the techniques that didn't use the heart-lung machine had fewer complications; there were lower rates of stroke, short-term memory loss, and bleeding; also, fewer patients needed blood transfusions, and hospital stays were shorter.

Off-pump bypass now accounts for 30 to 40 percent of the bypasses performed in the United States. It's often considered the safest approach for people seventy-five years of age and older, a group that's more at risk for stroke. The presence of plaque in the aorta may signal a higher risk for stroke, in which case an off-pump technique may be a better choice. Though off-pump techniques are gaining favor, studies are still going on to determine who is best suited for off-pump bypass.

At a few centers, surgeons are attempting another less invasive surgery called *port-access coronary artery bypass* or *PACAB*. Here, the surgeon makes small holes (ports) in the chest and inserts instruments through them; a tiny video camera feeds pictures to a video monitor, and the surgeon performs the operation by watching the monitor. Arteries from the chest or veins from the legs are used to bypass clogged heart vessels. This technique requires that the heart be stopped and blood gets pumped through the heart-lung machine.

Robotic surgery is another newer technique that is being

studied. It holds some promise but is limited in the scope of the operation that can be performed.

Hybrid Approaches

Another newer alternative to traditional bypass surgery is the *hybrid coronary bypass*, sometimes called *hybrid revascularization*. The hybrid approach combines the MIDCAB or OPCAB procedure with stenting. In this combined procedure, a cardiac surgeon performs the bypass operation and an interventional cardiologist performs the angioplasty.

The timing of the procedures depend on the narrowings. Until recently, if you needed both procedures, you would undergo two separate operations. If both procedures are being performed at the same time, there's greater convenience and less stress involved. Most patients can go home in few days. When staged, the clinical situation will determine the order of the procedures. The best candidates for the hybrid approach have:

- blockage in the left anterior descending (LAD) artery, requiring bypass
- additional blockages in non-LAD arteries that can be treated with stents

This newer hybrid approach is still being evaluated in selected patients, but has shown great promise and is being used more frequently.

Other alternative techniques that initially seemed promising have fallen short of expectations. One of these technologies is *transmyocardial revascularization (TMR)*. This procedure involves drilling holes in the heart muscle in an attempt to stimulate the growth of new vessels. Randomized trials did not show a benefit over standard heart medications. TMR is still being used for some patients with severe angina who cannot be treated with either CABG or angioplasty.

Hope for the Future

Angiogenesis

The growth of new blood vessels, called *angiogenesis*, is a naturally occurring process in the body. When your body is injured, these new vessels help restore blood flow to the injured tissues. Researchers are trying to harness the power of angiogenesis to stimulate blood vessel growth and enhance blood flow in cardiac patients. Studies of therapeutic angiogenesis are ongoing.

Stem Cell Muscle Repair and Regeneration

Stem cell research represents a new frontier in treating a damaged heart. Researchers are currently exploring ways that stem cells can help a diseased or damaged heart regain its pumping power. Early research results show that a variety of stem cells may be able to restore partially function to a diseased heart by replacing damaged heart muscle cells and establishing new blood vessels to supply them. Studies have shown improved heart function and healing of the damaged heart muscle when stem cells were injected soon after a heart attack. Newer studies demonstrate that stem cells may also be able to repair heart muscles several years after a heart attack.

9 Treating Coronary Heart Disease with Lifestyle Changes

Medical science has made great strides in treating coronary heart disease. As noted in chapter 7, new and better medications are more effective and have fewer side effects. Surgical interventions are more sophisticated than ever, leading to fewer complications and better outcomes. However, heart authorities, including the American Heart Association, agree that changing unhealthful lifestyle habits is still the single most important thing you can do to prevent coronary heart disease and stop it from progressing. There's evidence that making heart-healthy lifestyle changes, such as changing what you eat, your activity level, and how you deal with stress, may prevent a heart attack and may even reverse the narrowing of your arteries.

Lower Your High Blood Cholesterol

As you know, having high blood cholesterol is a major risk factor for CHD and heart attack. High levels of "bad" LDL cholesterol and triglycerides and low levels of "good" HDL cholesterol play a major role in the development of CHD and heart attacks.

If you have high cholesterol, your doctor will likely recommend changes in your diet and other lifestyle modifications. You may also need to take cholesterol-lowering medication.

You can control several things that affect your blood cholesterol:

- What you eat. If you're eating a lot of saturated fat, dietary cholesterol, and too many calories (leading to excess weight), chances are you have high cholesterol.
- Weight. Being overweight can make your "bad" LDL cholesterol go up and your "good" HDL cholesterol go down.
- Physical activity. Being inactive makes you a candidate for high LDL and low HDL.

Adopt a Heart-Healthy Diet

A *heart-healthy diet* is an integral part of getting your high blood cholesterol under control. Research has shown that a heart-healthy diet can slow the progression of plaque and also stabilize and even reverse atherosclerosis. Dietary changes can reduce total and LDL cholesterol levels by 10 to 15 percent, which translates to as much as a 20 to 30 percent reduction in heart disease risk.

If you're like most Americans, your diet contains 35 to 45 percent fat and 400 to 500 milligrams per day of cholesterol. That's way too much fat and cholesterol for a healthy heart. In Japan, where people eat a low-fat diet that typically contains 10 to 20 percent fat, CHD and high blood cholesterol are rare.

Eat less total dietary fat. The American Heart Association (AHA) recommends getting no more than 30 percent of your total daily calories from fat. The National Cholesterol Education Program

(NCEP) of the National Institutes of Health recommends 25 to 35 percent of your total calories come from fat.

Eat less saturated fat. Saturated fat is the biggest culprit in raising blood cholesterol, especially "bad" LDL cholesterol. Saturated fats come from animal products, such as meat and dairy products, and from tropical oils, such as palm and coconut oils. The NCEP recommends that you get up to 10 percent of your daily fat calories from saturated fats; the AHA has lowered its recommendation to no more than 7 percent.

Eat less trans fats. Along with saturated fats, trans fats raise LDL cholesterol levels. Trans fat comes from a process called *hydrogenation*, in which manufacturers add hydrogen to vegetable oil to increase the shelf life and flavor stability of their foods. Trans fat is commonly found in hard margarine, shortening, french fries, and commercial snack foods like cookies, crackers, cakes, and pies. Check food labels, which now include a listing of trans fat grams, and cut back on products containing partially hydrogenated oils. Use soft margarine and liquid vegetable oils rather than hard margarine or shortening.

Eat some unsaturated fats. When it comes to the heart, not all fats are created equal. Polyunsaturated fats (safflower, sesame, sunflower, corn, and soybean oil, and oils from nuts) and monounsaturated fats (olive, canola, peanut, and avocado oils) are made from vegetable sources. Both types may lower blood cholesterol when used in place of saturated fats. Monounsaturated fat, in particular, has been associated with lowering LDL cholesterol.

The AHA recommends up to 10 percent of your fat calories come from polyunsaturated fats and up to 15 percent from monounsaturated fat. New guidelines from NCEP recommend up to 10 percent polyunsaturated fat calories and up to 20 percent monounsaturated fat calories.

Limit dietary cholesterol. Dietary cholesterol is found in foods from animals (meat, fish, poultry, eggs, and dairy products). These foods are also sources of saturated fat. Egg yolks and organ meats like liver are loaded with cholesterol. One egg contains 215 milligrams of cholesterol, whereas egg whites contain none. Foods from plant sources such as fruits, vegetables, grains, cereals, nuts, and seeds contain no cholesterol. A 3½ ounce portion of shrimp contains 195 milligrams of cholesterol, whereas 3½ ounces of canned tuna (when packed in water) contain 30 milligrams of cholesterol.

The AHA recommends limiting dietary cholesterol to no more than 300 milligrams per day for men and 220 to 260 milligrams per day for women. For those who've had a coronary event, the AHA recommends less than 200 milligrams per day. The NCEP also recommends no more than 200 milligrams per day.

Choose foods high in complex carbohydrates. Foods that are high in carbohydrates (starches and sugars), such as rice, pasta, and potatoes, are loaded with vitamins and minerals and are actually lower in calories than high-fat foods. The AHA recommends that carbohydrates make up 55 to 60 percent of the calories in your daily diet. The NCEP recommendation is also for 50 to 60 percent carbohydrates.

The American Diabetes Association reports that more patients lose weight when they follow a lower carbohydrate diet—one made up of 45 to 50 percent carbohydrates and 30 to 35 percent fat. Individuals following this diet lost more weight than those following a conventional calorie-restricted diet made up of 55 to 60 percent carbohydrates and less than 30 percent fat.

Eat to Lower Cholesterol Levels

Eat foods rich in fiber. The indigestible parts of plant foods, fiber can help lower cholesterol and help keep you "regular." Some studies indicate eating fiber-rich foods may lower blood cholesterol. Additionally, fiber may be instrumental in preventing colon cancer, hemorrhoids, and the development of painful, saclike pouches (diverticula) in the intestine. It also makes you feel fuller, which can help prevent overeating. Fiber is found in fresh fruits and vegetables and whole grains. The AHA suggests getting plenty of fiber by eating five to nine servings per day of fruits and vegetables and six or more servings of grain products, including whole grains. The NCEP recommends eating twenty to thirty grams of fiber each day.

Choose lean protein. Limit protein to no more than six ounces per day and choose leaner cuts of meat, chicken, and fish instead of fatty meats. Beans, legumes, and soy products such as tofu are good, low-fat sources of protein. Choose fat-free, 1 percent fat, or low-fat dairy products.

Choose foods low in salt. A diet low in sodium can be helpful in reducing the risk of heart disease, stroke, and kidney disease. Choosing foods that are low in salt can also reduce high-blood pressure. Sodium is a common ingredient in many canned foods, condiments, and frozen foods. Look for labels that say "low-sodium" and compare labels when shopping. When cooking, replace salt with herbs and spices or salt-free seasoning mixes.

Balance calorie intake with output. Don't overeat. Eating more calories than you burn leads to becoming overweight, a major risk factor for CHD and heart attack.

Limit alcohol. Drinking a small amount of alcohol is associated with fewer heart-related problems. However, most heart authorities don't recommend taking up drinking alcohol if you don't drink. Alcohol abuse is associated with increases in a number of health problems, including high blood pressure and an elevation in triglycerides (both are CHD risk factors). If you do enjoy an occasional drink, limit your intake to no more than two alcoholic drinks per day for men, one per day for women.

Limit food and beverages with added sugars. Many snack foods and beverages contain added sugars that increase calorie intake. These foods and beverages are generally lacking in vitamins and minerals and can make you hungrier, causing you to consume even more calories. Be sure to read the labels of foods and beverages you buy and avoid products with these added sugars: sucrose, fructose, glucose, dextrose, corn syrup, maltose, high-fructose corn syrup, concentrated fruit juice, and honey.

How Much Fat Should You Eat?

The American Heart Association's guidelines for the amount of fat calories you should consume to follow their food plan call for 30 percent of one's daily calories to come from fat and 7 percent from saturated fat. The table below lists the amount of fat you can consume daily under this plan.

Total Daily Calories	Fat Calories Allowed	Saturated Fat Calories Allowed
1,500	450 (50 grams)	105 (12 grams)
1,800	540 (60 grams)	126 (14 grams)
2,000	600 (67 grams)	140 (16 grams)
2,500	750 (83 grams)	175 (19 grams)

Note: Each gram of fat equals 9 calories

Other Diet Plans

The AHA's eating plan and the NCEP's dietary recommendations aren't the only heart-healthy diets you can follow. Let's look at a few of the more popular heart-healthy diets.

Mediterranean-Style Diets

Studies have associated Mediterranean-style diets with a lower risk of heart disease. In general, fewer people from the Mediterranean countries of Spain, Greece, and Italy die from CHD than people in northern Europe or the United States.

Since diets vary among peoples of the Mediterranean countries and even among regions within countries, there's no single diet we can label the *Mediterranean diet*. Generally speaking, Mediterranean diets are rich in fruits, vegetables, cereals, fish, and beans. Mediterranean diets are also higher in total fat than other heart-healthy diets. However, the fats are primarily monounsaturated (mostly olive oil) and omega-3 fats, those found in cold-water fish such as herring, salmon, tuna, and mackerel and in soybean and canola oils.

The Mediterranean-style diet is heart healthy because it contains a number of protective nutrients: antioxidants such as vitamin E from fruits and vegetables, monounsaturated fatty acids from olive oil, and polyunsaturated omega-3 fatty acids from fish. Studies have shown that monounsaturated and polyunsaturated fats may make platelets (clotting elements in the blood) less sticky and therefore less likely to clot. For diabetics, these fats (when substituted for saturated fats) can also help lower blood cholesterol better than the higher carbohydrate containing diets advocated by the AHA and NCEP.

Asian Diet

Like the Mediterranean-style diet, there is no single Asian diet. However, research shows that Asians who eat a traditional diet have low rates of chronic disease, including CHD. That's because most Asian cuisine emphasizes plant-based foods, including vegetables, rice, beans, soy foods, nuts, seeds, and tea. The traditional Asian diet is low in fat; includes moderate amounts of fish, poultry, and eggs; and is low in red meats, cheese, and yogurt. In fact, in many Asian countries, traditional cuisine doesn't include dairy products at all.

Ornish Diet

Dean Ornish, M.D., director of the Preventive Medicine Research Institute in Sausalito, California, and author of *Dr. Dean Ornish's Program for Reversing Heart Disease*, published studies in the early 1990s showing that a comprehensive program of very low-fat, vegetarian eating; regular exercise; and stress management can actually *reverse* atherosclerosis in some patients with heart disease. Overall, Dr. Ornish found that the plaque in patients who adhered to less stringent diets (such as those advocated by the AHA and NCEP) continued to increase. Those on the AHA and NCEP diets experienced more than twice as many coronary events as those on the Ornish program.

The Ornish Diet, also called the "Reversal Diet," is a vegetarian diet that restricts total fat to 10 percent. It emphasizes fruits, vegetables, beans, whole grains, and nonfat dairy products and contains no meat, fish, poultry, or added fat.

Dr. Ornish's research has shown that over time even severe atherosclerosis can be reversed without the use of drugs in some patients. While a very low-fat vegetarian diet may not be right for everyone, Ornish's diet offers an alternative for reducing CHD risk.

Low-Carbohydrate Diets

Diets that restrict the carbohydrates, such as the South Beach, Atkins, and Zone plans, have become very popular, but they remain controversial. Low-carb diets are based on the theory that carbohydrate consumption increases insulin levels, which prompts the body to store fats instead of burn them. In turn, this leads to obesity and its complications, such as heart disease. These diets claim that limiting carbohydrate intake reduces insulin levels, causing the body to burn fat. By reducing obesity and fat, the risk of CHD is lowered.

Although these various diets limit carbohydrates, they differentiate among carbohydrates. For example, vegetables are viewed as a better option than sugar, grains, and starches. The many low-carb diets also differ from each other in the proportions of carbohydrates, protein, and fat they recommend.

The heart healthiness of these diets continues to be debated in the medical community. No long-term studies have been done but several short-term, independent clinical trials have reported improvements in cholesterol levels and lowered risk for heart disease. However, critics argue that replacing carbohydrates with protein and fat can lead to higher consumption of cholesterol and saturated fats, both of which have been proven to increase the risk of CHD.

One key tip if you choose a low-carb diet: avoid food with saturated fats, which can contribute to high cholesterol levels.

Tailoring a diet to your individual needs makes sense. Seek out a dietary professional for a consultation.

Lose Excess Weight

Being overweight isn't just a cosmetic problem. It is a risk factor for CHD, diabetes, high blood cholesterol, high triglycerides, and high blood pressure. Carrying excess weight puts a strain on your heart, making it work harder, even at rest. It also increases total cholesterol, "bad" LDL cholesterol, and triglycerides and decreases "good" HDL cholesterol, all contributing to the buildup of atherosclerotic plaque. If you carry your extra weight around your waist, the risk to your heart is even greater. It's no wonder the American Heart Association calls excessive weight a major risk factor for heart disease.

Losing even a small amount—5 to 10 percent—of your body weight can help decrease your risks. Losing as little as eleven to twenty-two pounds can decrease your risk of developing high blood pressure by as much as 25 percent. It can also help lower your "bad" LDL cholesterol and triglycerides and increase your "good" HDL cholesterol.

The How-to of Losing Weight

Work with your doctor. Have a checkup before you begin a weight-loss program. Your doctor can help you develop a sensible weight-loss program.

Set a reasonable goal. Your initial weight loss goal should be 10 percent of your current weight. Once you achieve this goal, set another goal, if needed.

Allow enough time. Slow and steady is the best path to permanent weight loss. Six months is a reasonable timeline for losing

10 percent of your current weight.

Aim for one to two pounds per week. Most women can lose one to two pounds a week by eating 1,200 to 1,500 calories per day. Most men can lose this amount by eating 1,500 to 1,800 calories per day. Talk with your doctor about the right amount of calories per day for you.

Accept responsibility. You are the only one who can make changes in your diet and exercise regimen to lose weight. Are you ready to accept personal responsibility and reduce your risk for heart disease?

Cut the calories. Gram for gram, fat contains more than twice the calories of protein or carbohydrates (nine calories/gram for fat; four calories/gram for protein and carbohydrates). That's why cutting dietary fat cuts calories. Limiting processed carbs and starches is also very helpful for weight reduction.

Every calorie counts. Eating only 50 excess calories per day results in 5 pounds of weight gain a year.

Choose a balanced approach. Follow the low-saturated-fat, low-calorie guidelines in this chapter. Choose nutrient-rich, low-calorie foods such as raw vegetables, some fruits, and complex carbohydrates (rice, pasta, whole-grain breads and cereals).

Avoid crash or fad diets. They may promise quick results, but they don't promote lifestyle changes that will enable you to maintain weight loss for a lifetime.

Take a multivitamin. Take a daily vitamin and mineral supplement to ensure you're meeting the minimum daily requirements.

Drink plenty of water. Drinking six to eight glasses of water a day is not only good for you, it'll help fill you up.

Keep a diary. Recording everything you eat can help you avoid deviating from your plan. Also, use your diary to record your weight loss, how you're feeling, and your exercise routine.

Weigh yourself once per week. Weighing yourself every day may be discouraging. The changes usually reflect only fluctuations in water retention.

Watch for danger zones. All of us have food triggers—people, places, and things that make us want to overeat or indulge in high-fat, high-calorie foods. Identify and avoid your food triggers and always think about portion control.

Slow down. It takes fifteen minutes or so after eating for your brain to "register" fullness signals. Slow down and take your time. Eating lots of high-fiber foods like vegetables can also make you feel fuller.

Reward yourself. As you achieve mini-goals in your weight-loss plan, reward yourself with small, non-food rewards (e.g., take yourself to a movie, buy a music CD or book).

Exercise. A program of regular exercise can help you eat less, increase the calories you burn, and help reduce other CHD risk factors. It can also decrease abdominal fat, the most dangerous type. Regular exercise is key to maintaining weight loss. Exercise experts say that for weight loss, how hard you exercise isn't as important as for how long. For instance, the calorie expenditure per unit time of exercise varies according to how rigorous the exercise is.

As you lose fat and your body becomes more efficient at using calories, you'll need to increase how much you exercise to lose further body fat. For the most effective weight loss, start by walking thirty minutes (or build up to thirty minutes) three times a week. Over time, build up to forty-five minutes a day at least five times a week. Your permanent exercise/weight-management goal should be to exercise at least thirty minutes or more a day most (preferably all) days of the week.

Exercise Regularly

As noted previously, regular exercise is key to reducing high blood cholesterol and losing and keeping off excess weight. Physical inactivity is clearly a risk factor for heart disease. By exercising regularly, you can cut your risk of having a heart attack by nearly 50 percent. Even if you've already had a heart attack, regular physical activity can lower the risk of having a second one. Regular exercise:

- Lowers blood pressure and helps prevent the development of high blood pressure. If you have mild high blood pressure and you exercise, your blood pressure will drop to healthier levels for eight to twelve hours after exercising. In some individuals, regular exercise is as effective as medication for lowering high blood pressure—without negative side effects.
- Lowers heart rate, allowing the heart to pump more efficiently. Exercise also helps reduce dangerous swings in heart rate.
- Improves blood cholesterol. Exercise can drop your total blood cholesterol by as much as 24 percent and "bad" LDL cholesterol by 10 percent. Exercise can also increase "good" HDL cholesterol by as much as 6 percent. The amount of activity needed for these improvements is moderate (e.g. a thirty-minute walk most days of the week).
- Lowers the body's tendency to produce dangerous blood

clots, a key factor in heart attack and stroke. Regular exercise raises the levels of plasminogen, an anticoagulant that may help prevent blood clots.

- Burns body fat. As you know, excess fat is a risk factor for heart disease, high blood pressure, diabetes, and other serious health problems. Exercise helps the body use insulin more efficiently and burn fat. It also helps the body clear excess sugar from the blood and makes it more sensitive to insulin, reducing the risk of diabetes.
- Reduces stress, a potential contributor to heart disease risk.

Is It Safe to Exercise?

For most people, even those with heart disease, the health benefits of exercise far outweigh the risks. One study published in the journal *Circulation* found elderly men aged seventy-one to ninety-three cut their risk of heart attack by 50 percent simply by walking about two miles a day. Another study found that people who exercised following a heart attack lowered their risk of having a second attack by 60 percent.

However, if you have a chronic health condition or other serious health problem, your doctor may want to outline some special exercise precautions. See your doctor for a pre-exercise checkup if you:

- have heart or lung disease, arthritis, or kidney disease
- have CHD risk factors (smoking, high blood pressure, diabetes, etc.)
- are taking medicine for high blood pressure or a heart condition

- are age forty or older
- are overweight
- have a family history of early CHD

If you have heart disease, your doctor may want you to undergo an exercise stress test to determine how much exercise is safe for you. It can help you know what maximum heart rate during exercise is safe for you (you can monitor your heart rate during exercise with a pulsemeter). For those who've had a heart attack or undergone angioplasty/stent or bypass surgery, your doctor should prescribe cardiac rehabilitation, which features carefully supervised physical activity.

The most common risk of physical activity is joint or muscle injury. This usually happens when you start exercising too hard or for too long, especially if you haven't been active for some time. Most of these injuries can be prevented by warming up before and cooling down after exercise and building up stamina slowly.

Heat exhaustion or heatstroke can be another problem if you're exercising during hot, humid weather. Both can be avoided with a little common sense—drink plenty of water, exercise less intensely on hot days, try to exercise during a cooler time of day, and watch for warning signs such as dizziness, headache, and nausea.

Rarely, people have died while exercising. This can be a big fear for someone who has heart disease. For people who have heart disease, following your doctor's orders and gradually building up your condition will reduce the risk of exercise-related problems. If you're considered high risk for heart attack, you should exercise in a monitored facility with staff who are trained in cardiac resuscitation.

How to Make Exercise a Success

Go slowly. Start slowly and build up. If you're inactive, you may want to begin with a ten to fifteen-minute walk, three times a week. Over time, increase the time and speed.

Warm up, cool down. Allow five minutes or so of stretching and slow movement to allow your body to prepare for exercise. After working out, spend another five minutes exercising slowly to cool down.

Listen to your body. Don't exercise through pain. At first, you may feel a little stiff after exercising. But you shouldn't feel pain. If you hurt a joint, or pull a muscle or tendon, stop the activity for several days. Most minor injuries can be healed with RICE—*r*est, *i*ce, *c*ompression, and *e*levation—and over-the-counter painkillers.

Keep the pace. To condition your heart and lungs, you need to exercise at a brisk enough pace to make you breathe deeply and sweat a bit. However, you still should be able to carry on a conversation.

Watch for warning signs. Stop activity and call your doctor immediately if you experience any of these symptoms: sudden dizziness, cold sweat, paleness, fainting, and/or pain or pressure in your chest during or after exercising.

Pay attention to the weather. Exercise indoors on a hot day, or outdoors during cooler parts of the day. Wear loose, lightweight clothing and drink lots of water before, during, and after exercising. During colder weather, layer clothing and wear a hat.

Stay with it. Make exercise a priority. Schedule time for it and put it on your calendar. Ask a friend to be an exercise buddy. Join an exercise class. Choose activities you like and that you'll stick with.

Have patience. It'll take time to get into better shape. Fitness experts say a program of moderate activity like brisk walking three times a week will improve the functioning of your heart and blood vessels within eight to ten weeks. If you exercise four times weekly, improvement can be seen within three to four weeks.

Lower Your High Blood Pressure

Nearly one in four Americans has high blood pressure (HBP). Also called hypertension, HBP occurs when small arteries (arterioles) become constricted, which makes it difficult for blood to pass through them. This forces the heart to work harder, straining both the heart and the arteries. As the heart works harder, over time, it can enlarge. If the heart becomes sufficiently enlarged, it may be unable to pump enough blood to the body (a condition called heart failure). Organs denied the blood and oxygen they need can't work properly. HBP can also cause the arteries and arterioles to become scarred and less elastic, which makes them prime candidates for artery-clogging atherosclerosis.

How to Lower Your Blood Pressure

Obviously, you can't do anything about your gender, family history, age, race, or preexisting health conditions, all of which can influence your blood pressure. However, you can lose weight. As mentioned earlier, being overweight is a major risk factor for high blood pressure. In fact, experts estimate that 75 percent of all high blood pressure is related to excessive weight. These lifestyle changes will lower your blood pressure:

- Lose excess weight.
- Limit alcohol.
- Limit caffeine intake.

- Exercise regularly.
- Limit your salt intake.
- Get enough potassium, calcium, and magnesium.
- Stop smoking.

Limit Salt Intake

Not everyone is "salt sensitive"; however, if you have high blood pressure, your doctor will likely want you to restrict the salt in your diet. For many people, the amount of table salt (sodium chloride) they consume affects their blood pressure. People who have hypertension or diabetes, or who are older tend to be more sensitive to dietary salt.

The average American consumes about 4,000 to 6,000 milligrams of salt every day—too much for good heart health. Most people should consume no more than 2,400 milligrams of salt a day—about one teaspoon; however, doctors will recommend that some people with heart conditions avoid even this much salt.

There are three other minerals you should be concerned about if you have high blood pressure: potassium, calcium, and magnesium. Deficiencies in all three are associated with high blood pressure. The following are suggestions for reducing dietary sodium while still getting enough potassium, calcium, and magnesium.

Follow the DASH diet plan. This plan, the "Dietary Approaches to Stop Hypertension," provides good guidelines, intended to lower blood pressure, reduce cholesterol, and improve the way in which your body uses insulin. You can learn more about this popular plan at www.dashdiet.org.

Keep a salt diary. Write down what you eat and how much sodium each food contains.

Don't add salt. Put away the salt shaker and avoid adding salt during cooking.

Avoid salty snacks. Plenty of foods are obviously loaded with salt—pretzels, chips, salt bagels, pickles, soy sauce, and cured foods. Choose lower-salt foods.

Look out for medicines with sodium. Some medicines, especially over-the-counter varieties like antacids, are loaded with sodium.

Limit processed foods. As much as 75 percent of the salt in American diets comes from processed foods. Opt for fresh, fresh frozen, or canned foods with no added salt.

Check labels. Nutrition labels list the amount of sodium. Watch out for ingredients such as sodium chloride, salt, MSG, and baking powder. Select for labels that say "low sodium," "no salt," "light sodium," "no added salt," etc. Rinse canned foods. Choose lower-sodium versions of canned products. Rinse the food with fresh water before using to minimize the salt content.

Eat potassium-rich foods. You need at least 3,500 milligrams of potassium per day, which you can get in a balanced, heart-healthy diet. Include plenty of fresh fruits and vegetables such as peaches, figs, bananas, apricots, lima beans, potatoes, spinach, sweet potatoes, and winter squash. Other foods high in potassium include fish, nuts, low-fat milk products, dried beans and peas, and whole-grain cereals. Note: if you have kidney disease or high blood potassium, consult your doctor about eating these foods.

Include sources of calcium. You need at least 1,200 milligrams of calcium per day for good health. Include skim or low-fat dairy products (lower-fat varieties have even more calcium than full-fat dairy products). If milk products upset your stomach, try lactose-free dairy products such as lactose-reduced or lactose-free milk.

Eat plenty of magnesium-rich foods. These include whole grains, leafy green vegetables, nuts, seeds, and dried peas and beans. *Caution*: If you have kidney problems, talk with your doctor about eating these foods.

Stop Smoking

Quitting smoking is one of the most important things you can do for your heart—and for your overall health. Smoking causes more than 400,000 deaths per year in the United States. It's a major cause of CHD and heart attack. Smoking causes as many as 30 percent of the CHD-related deaths in the United States each year and magnifies other CHD risk factors, multiplying the risk. In fact, if you smoke, you're two to six times more likely to have a heart attack compared with nonsmokers. Smokers who have heart attacks are more likely to die than nonsmokers. Smoking:

- reduces the ability of the blood to carry oxygen
- raises "bad" LDL cholesterol
- decreases "good" HDL cholesterol
- damages the lining of the coronary arteries, making them more vulnerable to plaque
- makes the blood coagulate more easily, increasing the risk of blood clots
- may trigger coronary spasm
- may lead to irregular heart rhythms

In addition, cigarette smoking is the biggest risk for *peripheral vascular disease*, narrowing of the blood vessels in the arms and legs. It also increases the risk for several types of cancer, chronic lung diseases, asthma, infertility, and impotence.

Quitting smoking can dramatically lower your risk for heart disease and other health problems, no matter how long you've smoked. The risk to your heart drops soon after you quit. Within two years of quitting smoking, your chances of dying from a heart attack will be cut in half. In ten years, your risk will be nearly the same as for someone who has never smoked (depending on your other risk factors).

> People with CHD who've had a heart attack and stop smoking cut their risk of another heart attack, sudden cardiac death, and dying from CHD by 50 percent.

The How-to's of Quitting Smoking

Recognize why you want to quit. Before you take the plunge, write down all the reasons you want to quit. Then write down all the benefits you'll receive as a nonsmoker, such as saving money, improved health, and cleaner-smelling clothing. Post your list where you'll see it every day. When you're tempted to smoke, review your list.

Talk with your doctor about medical help. You don't have to rely on willpower alone. Your doctor can prescribe nicotine replacement products (patches or gum) to ease your transition to nonsmoking. Nicotine replacements deliver small, steady doses of nicotine without the "buzz" that keeps you hooked. While they contain nicotine, they don't deliver the tar and carbon monoxide responsible for some of the adverse health effects of smoking. An even newer option is the "anti-smoking pill," *Zyban* (*bupropion hydrochloride*), which contains no nicotine but appears to affect chemicals in the brain associated with nicotine addiction. Combined with behavior modification, both nicotine replacement products and Zyban have proven successful for many smokers.

A newer drug, *varenicline*, which is sold as Chantix, is also available for smoking cessation. Chantix has been shown to have abstinence rates of more than 40 percent in twelve-week studies. Approximately 10 percent of users reported nausea, headache, insomnia, and unusual dreams. However, rarely did these side effects require discontinuation of the drug.

Set a quit date. Mark it on your calendar. Then stick to it.

Prepare your environment. Toss out all cigarettes, ashtrays, lighters, and matches you may have in your home, workplace, or car. Wash your curtains, bedclothes, and anything else that has cigarette smoke odor. Make your environment off-limits to cigarette smoking. Secondhand smoke is also a major risk factor.

Enlist the support of others. Tell your friends and family you're quitting. Ask them to help.

Recognize and avoid your triggers. Certain situations, people, and places can make you want to smoke. Take time to list all your triggers. Then avoid them.

Be prepared for withdrawal. Know that you're going to experience some unpleasant sensations when you quit—headache, anxiety, nervousness, cravings, etc. But even people who have smoked for years overcome withdrawal symptoms within two to four weeks. Some people have successfully used acupuncture or hypnosis to combat these symptoms. Others prefer to use temporary nicotine replacement products to lessen withdrawal.

Drink large quantities of water and fruit juices. They will help wash the nicotine out of your body.

Change behaviors. If, for instance, you smoke right after a meal, take a walk instead. If you smoke while driving, carpool with nonsmokers or take the bus.

Exercise. Take up walking, biking, or any other physical activity you enjoy. It'll help you combat the stress of quitting and help your heart and lungs recover.

Learn to relax. Try deep breathing. Take long, deep breaths. Repeat at least five times. Learn to meditate. Listen to relaxation audiotapes or soothing music.

Keep your hands busy. Sew, crochet, carve wood, do crossword puzzles, garden, write letters.

Record and reward your progress. As you reach each new milestone—one week, one month, two months, six months, a year—mark it on the calendar and then do something nice to reward yourself.

Keep a savings bank. Put in it the money you're saving each day from not smoking. Plan to do something wonderful (like take a trip) with the savings.

Don't have "just one." Weeks or months after you quit, don't think you can have "just one" cigarette without getting hooked again.

Get back on the horse. If you smoke after you've quit, don't punish yourself. Just review your reasons for quitting and start again.

10   Alternative Treatments

At this point, you may be saying, "Yes, but aren't there alternatives for me? What about meditation or taking vitamins or herbal supplements? I've heard about alternative ways to clean out the arteries. What about those?" Let's look at what some of the research says about other types of treatment for coronary heart disease. One of these treatments is known as *integrative medicine*; it is an approach that encourages the patient to participate in their own healing. Symptoms that integrative medicine can address include: stress, anxiety, pain, insomnia, depression, and side effects from anesthesia and medications.

Stress Management

Do stress and personality traits cause CHD and subsequent heart attacks? This question is still being hotly debated. Much of the research indicates that one's response to stress and the traits of hard-driving personality types (so-called type A's) can increase the risk of heart disease. We don't know if it's how stress influences the body directly or whether it's the unhealthy responses

to it (smoking, overeating, drinking, inactivity)—or a combination—that increases CHD risk. Whatever the cause, doctors do know that psychological stress can trigger:

- increases in blood pressure
- rapid heart rate
- narrowing of arteries
- chest pain
- activation of clotting agents in the blood
- release of fats into the bloodstream
- release of the hormone *cortisol*, which raises blood cholesterol
- dangerous heart rhythm disturbances (arrhythmias)

What exactly is stress? It's a term used to describe a person's response to physical, emotional, and environmental factors. It's *not* the events or people or situations that frighten, enrage, or annoy us that cause stress. It's our *reaction* to them. All of us know people who just seem to serenely go through life. Things never seem to faze them. Then there are others who react—or overreact—to the least little inconvenience or disappointment with anger, hostility, worry, anxiety, depression, and other unhealthy emotions. One study published in the journal *Circulation* found that people who frequently feel depressed are more likely to develop heart disease. Another found the risk of heart attack increases for at least two hours following an angry outburst. Still other studies suggest that a chronic state of stress can cause permanent increases in heart rate, blood pressure, and possibly blood cholesterol, all of which increase the risk of CHD and heart attack.

Most heart experts recommend a program of stress management as a part of an overall treatment plan for CHD. Here are some suggestions to de-stress your life:

Practice relaxation. A number of techniques are effective in helping people relax and unwind. Take a class to learn to meditate. Do yoga. Buy some progressive relaxation tapes. Ask your doctor for a referral to a qualified practitioner who can teach you biofeedback techniques. Also, try this deep-breathing exercise. Sit in a quiet, comfortable place where you won't be disturbed. Close your eyes. Take a deep breath in. At the top of your inhalation, hold for three to five seconds. Then slowly let your breath out, trying to make your exhalation longer than your inhalation. Use your stomach muscles to squeeze out all the air. Then take another deep inhalation, hold, and exhale. Repeat for five to six breaths.

Exercise regularly. Aerobic exercise that is rhythmic, uses the large muscles of the arms and legs, and makes you breathe deeply is an excellent stress reducer. Brisk walking, jogging, bicycling, and swimming are all good forms of aerobic exercise. This type of exercise stimulates *endorphins*—the same "feel good" chemicals that runners experience as the "runner's high." A brisk walk of 30 minutes per day can lower your systolic blood pressure by 4 to 9 points.

If you want to start an exercise program, follow these steps as outlined in the Mayo Clinic Fitness & Sports Medicine Center: 1) See your doctor, 2) Assess your fitness level, 3) Design your program (including stretching and cross-training), 4) Assemble your equipment (from sneakers to weights), 5) Get Started, and 6) Measure your progress.

Practice yoga. Yoga has been shown to increase relaxation and reduce stress and anxiety. In addition to yoga's calming effects, it improves strength and flexibility, which may in turn help control respiration, blood pressure, and heart and metabolic rates. One study has even found that practicing yoga can reduce cholesterol levels and slow the progression of heart disease. Because yoga's gentle stretches and poses can be modified to suit each individual's abilities, it can be performed by virtually anyone at any age.

Practice Tai Chi. Tai Chi is an ancient form of Chinese martial arts that incorporates gentle physical activity, meditation, and rhythmic breathing techniques. This increasingly popular activity has been found to reduce stress, lower blood pressure, and reduce the risk of heart disease. In older adults, it can also improve balance, posture, flexibility, strength, and stamina.

Get some rest. In this fast-paced world, too many of us are sleep deprived. Not getting enough sleep can leave you fatigued and vulnerable to stress. Most people need at least six to eight hours of sleep a night.

For a good night's sleep:

- Try to go to bed at the same time every night.
- Make your bedroom dark and quiet.
- Avoid caffeinated drinks and foods and exercising late in the day.
- Be careful about the television or radio programs you watch, especially right before going to bed (don't expect a restful night's sleep after watching stories on national or international crises on the news).

Prioritize. Many people feel stressed because their life is too busy. Learn to prioritize. List all the things you do and for each one ask yourself, Is this essential? Could someone else do it? Then delegate. Learn to say no to those demands that aren't critical.

Set aside "me" time. Few adults get time all to themselves, yet it's essential for good mental health and for keeping a lid on stress. Give yourself time every day—even if it's only a few minutes—to do something you really enjoy. Go out and pick flowers in your garden. Putter in your shop. Take up a hobby that interests you. Take a class in a subject you want to learn about. Other potentially helpful activities include music and art therapies as well as a massage.

Develop a support system. People who are socially isolated are at greater risk for serious health problems, including heart disease. Take the time to develop and maintain a group of close, supportive friends. Let your family and friends know you care about them.

Get organized. Nothing stresses like being late or disorganized. Get up fifteen minutes earlier or leave a few minutes sooner so that you're not rushing. Set your clothes out the night before. Make an effort to organize areas of your life that are a mess. Perhaps you need a file folder system to organize your bills. Or set up a hook system where you hang up your keys rather than having to rush around frantically looking for them. If you have trouble organizing yourself, there are plenty of organizing professionals who can help.

Volunteer. Nothing helps us get out of ourselves as well as helping someone less fortunate. It can provide a social outlet and possibly a new source of friends as well as the satisfaction of making a worthwhile contribution. Think about things you care about—the environment, older people, the disabled, children's issues, veterans' rights, animals, whatever. Then contact the appropriate organization in your community and ask how you can help.

Vitamins and Other Supplements

Can you prevent or treat CHD with vitamins or other supplements? It's an attractive thought and one that researchers have been studying.

Omega-3 Fatty Acids

Omega-3 fatty acids are typically found in fatty fish, such as tuna, salmon, albacore, and sardines, among others. They are also available in supplements. Clinical trials have shown that omega-3 fatty acids are beneficial to the heart whether you're healthy, at risk for CHD, or already have CHD. The ways that omega-3 fatty acids reduce the risk of heart disease are still being studied, but research to date has shown that they can:

- lower triglyceride levels
- reduce the risk of arrhythmias, which can lead to sudden cardiac death
- reduce the growth rate of plaque in the arteries
- lower blood pressure (slightly)

For healthy adults, the AHA recommends increasing omega-3 fatty acid intake through food, specifically by eating fatty fish twice a week. However, if you already have CHD or high triglycerides, supplements may be recommended in addition to including fish in your diet. The AHA recommends consulting with your physician before taking any omega-3 fatty acid supplements. Note: the FDA has approved the drug, *Omacor*, a purer omega-3 preparation to reduce triglyceride levels.

Antioxidants (Vitamins A, C, and E)

One group of vitamins—the antioxidants—have been attracting a lot of attention for their potential for helping the heart. When cells use oxygen, they produce by-products called free radicals. These free radicals damage cells in a process called *oxidation.* In heart disease, free radicals are believed to be involved in the oxidation of LDL cholesterol, which contributes to atherosclerotic plaque buildup and subsequent heart attacks. Antioxidants can help prevent damage to tissues from oxidation by neutralizing free radicals. Three antioxidants that have received the most attention from researchers are vitamin A, vitamin E, and vitamin C.

Studies on these vitamins have been disappointing and show no evidence that they can prevent heart attacks or atherosclerosis. Scientific evidence suggests that consuming antioxidant vitamins does not reduce the need to lower your blood pressure, lower cholesterol, and stop smoking cigarettes. However, studies have shown that eating more fruits and vegetables does lower heart disease risk. As a result, most heart authorities recommend getting the antioxidants your heart needs from foods rather than from pills. Make sure you eat a balanced diet with plenty of antioxidant-rich fruits and vegetables.

Folate/B Vitamins

The amino acid homocysteine is a natural by-product of the body's use of protein and one of the many building blocks of proteins. There have been studies showing an association between homocysteine levels and blocked arteries. It was thought that by lowering the homocysteine levels in the body with supplements of folic acid and vitamins B_6 and B_{12}, homocysteine's adverse effect could be reduced. This combination of vitamins was successful at lowering the levels of homocysteine, but did not reduce the person's cardiac risk. It is now thought that homocysteine is more a marker than a cause of heart disease and, therefore, these vitamin supplements are not recommended.

Elevated homocysteine levels can be lowered by reducing fat in the diet, eating plenty of fresh fruits and vegetables, and getting enough folic acid, vitamin B_6, and vitamin B_{12}. (The recommended daily allowance (RDA) is 400 micrograms for folic acid, two milligrams for B_6, and six micrograms for B_{12}.) A diet rich in these naturally occurring vitamins makes sense.

> Supplements can interfere or interact negatively with some drugs. Talk to your doctor before taking them.

Garlic Supplements

Since garlic does have some disease-fighting qualities, many people are gulping down garlic supplements in hopes that it will reduce heart disease. Studies conducted on animals have shown that garlic lowers the production of triglycerides and cholesterol in the liver. Evidence shows that garlic thins the blood and makes it less likely that clots will form. It may also help prevent and may even reverse the growth of arterial plaque. Short-term studies have shown modest benefit in LDL cholesterol levels in humans; however, long-term proof of benefit at reducing cardiovascular mortality is lacking.

There are also questions about the form of garlic and the dose that's safe and effective. Some authorities suggest that garlic supplements aren't as effective as the natural dietary form because the stomach breaks down the compound largely responsible for the heart-healthy benefits. Cooking garlic may also change the healthful compounds. Eating large amounts of garlic can cause anemia and irritation of the gastrointestinal tract as well as bad breath. Because there's little regulation of food supplements, there's also the problem of knowing if what's listed on the label is actually what's in the tablets. For now, eating fresh garlic in your meals is the best way to enjoy its possible benefits.

Fiber

As mentioned in chapter 9, fiber (the indigestible parts of plants) can also lower "bad" LDL cholesterol by 10 to 15 percent. To increase your fiber, eat plenty of fresh fruits and vegetables (including the edible skins), whole grains, beans, and peas. Adding fiber-rich foods such as oat bran to your breakfast is an easy way to increase your fiber intake. The American Heart Association recommends getting twenty to twenty-five grams of fiber per day for good heart health. Diets with high fiber content have also been shown to reduce the risk of colon cancer.

Soy

People in Asian countries, who have low levels of heart disease, consume large amounts of soy foods. Natural soy compounds (*isoflavones*) may act like hormones that regulate cholesterol levels. When soy protein is used in place of animal protein, it lowers blood cholesterol levels. Soy's greatest benefit may be that it replaces the intake of other proteins such as meat, which is loaded with cholesterol and saturated fat. Consuming seventeen to twenty-five grams of soy protein per day is safe and may contribute to lowering "bad" LDL cholesterol and lowering your risk of heart disease by eighteen to twenty-eight percent. A recent study by Reynolds and colleagues in *The American Journal of Cardiology* confirms the beneficial effects of soy protein after analyzing forty-one randomized trials.

Green and Black Tea

Research from Japan published in the *Journal of the American Medical Association* confirmed the beneficial effects of *green tea* in reducing cardiovascular mortality after following more than 40,000 patients. The largest effect was seen in stroke reduction, especially in women. Overall, people who drank at least one cup of green tea daily had a 26 percent reduction in all causes of death, including cardiovascular disease. (Cancer rates were not affected.)

Some evidence suggests that *black tea* may be good for maintaining healthy arteries. *Flavonoids* in black tea—and also found in onions, dark beer, red wine, and red grape juice—help prevent the oxidation of "bad" LDL cholesterol that leads to plaque. They also improve the function of the inner lining of the arteries, which respond to changes in the body's demands for oxygen and blood dilating or narrowing. When the lining is healthy, it's also better able to inhibit the formation of blood clots and inflammation of the vessel walls.

Red Wine

You've probably read stories suggesting that drinking red wine may protect against heart disease. The incidence of death from CHD in France, where they consume lots of red wine, is about half that of the United States, despite the fact that the French eat about the same amount of animal fat. Some believe this may be due to the antioxidant properties of flavonoids (also found in dark beer, red grape juice, onions, and black tea) and other compounds such as *resveratrol* in red wine. However, some studies show that it isn't just wine, but any type of distilled spirits that have this heart-protective effect.

Drinking alcohol in moderation (up to one drink a day for women, two for men) appears to lower the risk of heart attack. It also raises the levels of "good" HDL cholesterol and may help prevent blood clots.

Chelation Therapy

Used to treat atherosclerosis since the 1950s, *chelation therapy* involves thirty to fifty intravenous injections of *ethylenediamine-tetraacetic acid (EDTA)*. EDTA binds to minerals in the blood, including calcium, which are then excreted through the urine. Chelation is promoted as sort of a "drain cleaner" for the arteries, softening the plaques by removing the calcium in them. The lost minerals are replaced with oral supplements.

Chelation therapy is a proven therapy for removing heavy metals (such as lead) from the blood. However, no scientific studies prove that this expensive alternative therapy works for atherosclerosis. In a major randomized placebo controlled study involving 3,140 patients and published in the *Journal of the American Medical Association*, there was no benefit of chelation. Remember that the calcium measured by a CT scan is simply a *diagnostic marker* for CHD. The real problem with plaque is *not* necessarily the calcium, but the cholesterol at the core of the plaque. Medical authorities such as the American Heart Association, the American Medical Association, and the American College of Cardiology do not endorse chelation therapy for treating heart disease. A few years ago, the Food and Drug Administration, charging that chelation therapy has no scientific basis, took steps to prevent its proponents from making claims about its health benefits in treating heart disease.

Work with Your Doctor

Although current research doesn't indicate that most so-called alternative treatments for CHD really help, this doesn't mean that future studies won't find other treatments that are effective. In the meantime, it's important not to be taken in by false claims of unproven treatments or to use such treatments in place of ones that have been scientifically proven to work. Supplements, methods, or procedures that claim to be "secret" cures for heart disease aren't. There aren't secret cures in medicine.

Reputable medical research centers around the world are actively studying treatments for CHD, including many alternative treatments, such as supplements. Much of the research has resulted in newer, more effective medicines, diagnostic techniques, and treatment procedures like anigioplasty, stenting, and bypass surgery. In the future, CHD treatment will be even more effective. For now, it's important to work closely with your doctor to find the best treatments for you so that you can enjoy a long and healthy life.

Glossary

ACE inhibitors (ACEs): Also called angiotensin converting enzyme inhibitors, ACEs belong to a class of drugs used to lower high blood pressure and treat patients with heart failure and after heart attacks. ACEs block the formation of the chemical that causes tiny arteries to constrict.

Alpha-blockers: Blood pressure-lowering drugs that block the stimulation of specialized nerves.

Angina: The medical term is angina pectoris. Angina is chest pressure and pain caused when the heart doesn't receive enough oxygen.

AngioJet: A high-pressure spray device used with a catheter to break up blood clots.

Angioplasty: Also called balloon angioplasty or percutaneous transluminal coronary angioplasty (PTCA), angioplasty is an invasive procedure that treats the inside of coronary arteries without opening the chest.

Angiotensin: A chemical the body produces that causes small arteries (arterioles) to constrict.

Antiarrhythmics: Medications that correct heart rhythm problems.

Anticoagulants: Blood-thinning drugs that inhibit special proteins that form blood clots.

Antiplatelets: Drugs that reduce the ability of the blood to clot by inhibiting the normal function of platelets (blood clotting cells).

Aorta: The large artery that receives blood from the heart's left ventricle and carries it to the body.

Apoproteins: Proteins the body uses to coat cholesterol so that it can be transported in the blood.

ARBs: Also called angiotensin receptor blockers, these are drugs prescribed for high blood pressure. They block the chemical that causes tiny arteries to constrict.

Arrhythmia: Abnormal heartbeat.

Arterioles: Tiny arteries, the blood vessels that carry blood, oxygen, and nutrients to cells in the body.

Arteriosclerosis: Commonly called "hardening of the arteries," arteriosclerosis is a process in which the arteries become thicker and harder, losing their natural elasticity.

Artery: A blood vessel that carries blood away from the heart.

Atherosclerosis: A process in which deposits of cholesterol, cellular waste products, calcium, and other substances build up in the inner lining of arteries.

Atriums (or Atria): Top chambers of the heart.

Beta-blockers: A class of drugs often used to alleviate angina and treat high blood pressure. They block adrenaline's effect on the heart, decreasing heart rate, reducing the strength of the heart's contractions, and lowering blood pressure.

Blood pressure: A measurement of the force when the heart pumps blood into the arteries and out to the body, and the force of the arteries as they resist the blood from the heart. It's expressed in millimeters of mercury (mmHg).

Brachytherapy: Also called intracoronary radiation, brachytherapy involves exposing the arteries to gamma or beta radiation to reduce the incidence of arterial renarrowing.

Bruits: The rough, turbulent sounds of blood moving through narrowed arteries. Doctors use a stethoscope on the neck, abdomen, and elsewhere to detect bruits (French for noise).

Calcium channel blockers: Drugs that block or inhibit the movement of calcium in the heart, nerves, and blood vessel walls. These drugs reduce blood pressure and dilate coronary arteries.

Capillaries: Very small vessels, often too small to see, that connect the arterial and venous blood systems.

Cardiac angiography: Also called arteriography, angiocardiography, or cardiac catheterization and angiography, this invasive diagnostic technique uses flexible tubes called catheters threaded through the arteries. It can show blood flow problems and blockages in the coronary arteries.

Cardiac positron-emission tomography (PET): A nuclear imaging technology that can measure blood flow and metabolism in the heart.

Catheter: A long, slender, flexible tube used in angiography that is threaded through the arteries.

CAT scan: An imaging technique in which an X-ray beam is passed through the body as the scanner is rapidly rotated around the body. It produces a detailed cross section of the body.

Cholesterol: A waxy, fatlike substance that is found in every cell in the body. It is used to help digest fats, strengthen cell membranes, and make some types of hormones and vitamins. It is also a major component of plaque.

Coronary arteries: The arteries that branch from the aorta, divide into smaller arteries, and provide blood for the heart muscle.

Coronary artery bypass graft surgery (CABG): Surgery in which pieces of blood vessels are stitched around blocked arteries, creating bypasses around blockages.

Coronary heart disease (CHD): Also called coronary artery disease

(CAD) or ischemic heart disease, it is a condition caused when arteries become narrowed by plaque.

Coronary occlusion: Blockage of a coronary artery that restricts the blood supply.

Coronary thrombosis: Another name for coronary occlusion, a heart attack caused by a clot blocking blood supply to the heart.

Cyanotic: Skin that is bluish in color, which may be a sign of vascular disease or lack of oxygen.

Diabetes: Called diabetes mellitus, it's a disease in which the body isn't able to produce and/or respond to the hormone insulin, which converts blood sugar into energy.

Directional atherectomy: A procedure in which the cardiologist shaves away plaque and removes it from the body.

Dissection of the aorta: A life-threatening condition in which the inner lining of the major artery that leads away from the heart (aorta) becomes torn and may cause severe chest pain.

Diuretics: Drugs that flush excess water and sodium from the body by increasing urination.

Doppler ultrasound: Part of an echocardiogram study that produces heart sounds and displays a picture of the blood flowing between the chambers of the heart, and measures internal pressures.

Echocardiogram: A diagnostic test in which sound waves are used to "bounce back" images of the heart.

Electrocardiography (ECG): A diagnostic test that records the electrical activity of the heart.

Electron beam computed tomography (EBCT): This ultrafast CT scan detects CHD by measuring calcium in the blood vessels.

Endotracheal tube: A breathing tube used during bypass surgery.

Estrogen: A female hormone. Oral contraceptives and hormone replacement therapy (HRT) use synthetic forms of estrogen.

Exercise ECG: Also called a stress ECG or treadmill test, it's a diagnostic test that records the electrical activity of the heart under stress (exercise or medication).

Fibrates: Triglyceride-lowering medications.

Gene therapy: A new technology for treating disease, gene therapy involves introducing genetic material into cells to cause certain actions.

Heart attack: Also called myocardial infarction, a heart attack occurs when the blood supply to a portion of the heart muscle is blocked and the part of the heart that doesn't receive blood becomes damaged and dies.

Heart failure: A condition in which the heart becomes unable to pump efficiently and supply the body with the blood it needs.

High blood pressure: Also called hypertension, high blood pressure occurs when the blood pressure is 140/90 mm/Hg or higher, which strains the heart.

High-density lipoprotein: So-called "good" cholesterol, HDL cholesterol contains mostly protein. When there's excess cholesterol in the blood, HDL cholesterol picks up cholesterol deposited in the arteries and transports it to the liver for disposal.

Holter monitoring: Also called ambulatory ECG monitoring, it's a variation of electrocardiography that monitors and records the heart's electrical activity during everyday activities. It's used to detect heart problems that come and go.

Homocysteine: An amino acid that's a by-product of the body's use of protein. High levels of homocysteine have been associated with a low intake of folate, vitamin B_6, and vitamin B_{12} and is associated with heart disease.

Hydrogenation: A process used in making margarine and shortening in which unsaturated fats become more highly saturated fats.

In-stent restenosis: A condition in which arteries that are treated with stents (fine-mesh tubes) become renarrowed.

Insulin: A hormone produced by the pancreas that helps the body convert blood sugar (glucose) into a usable form for energy.

Internal mammary arteries (IMAs): Two arteries located on the inside chest wall that are often used in bypass surgery.

Intracoronary radiation: Also called brachytherapy, it's a procedure in which arteries treated with stents are exposed to radiation in an effort to stop or slow down the formation of scar tissue.

Intravascular ultrasound (IVUS): An imaging technology in which a small device mounted on the tip of a catheter is inserted into coronary arteries. The device sends back images of the inside of the arteries using ultrasound technology.

Ischemia: Reduced blood flow to an organ. In most cases, this reduction is caused by a blockage or narrowing of an artery.

Ischemic heart disease: Another name for coronary artery disease or coronary heart disease. Ischemic heart disease is caused by arteries becoming narrowed and causing a reduced blood supply to the heart.

Lipoprotein profile: A fasting blood test that measures total cholesterol, HDL and LDL cholesterol, and triglyceride levels. All adults should have a lipoprotein profile performed at least once every five years.

Lipoproteins: The protein "packages" that transport cholesterol in the blood.

Low-density lipoprotein: So-called "bad" cholesterol, LDL cholesterol contributes to plaque building in the arteries.

Magnetic Resonance Imaging (MRI): Formerly called nuclear magnetic resonance (NMR), this diagnostic test uses powerful magnets and radio waves to produce images of the inside of the body.

Myocardial infarction (MI): The medical term for heart attack. When blood supply to a part of the heart is severely reduced or blocked, a heart attack can occur. The area of the heart muscle on the other side of the blockage begins to die and results in permanent damage to the heart.

Nicotinic acid: The B vitamin niacin that's used to decrease LDL cholesterol and triglycerides and increase HDL cholesterol.

Nitrate: A type of anti-anginal medication used to widen the coronary arteries.

Nuclear scanning: A variety of diagnostic tests that involve injecting a tiny amount of radioactive material into the bloodstream and taking images of the radiation given off by the material.

Pericarditis: Inflammation of the fibrous sac that surrounds the heart (pericardium). The chest pain caused by pericarditis can mimic angina.

Plaque: A mixture of fatty substances, cholesterol, cellular waste products, calcium, and other substances that become deposited in the inner lining of arteries.

Platelets: The clotting cells in blood.

Pressure wire: A diagnostic tool used in the cath lab that measures pressures inside arteries to determine the significance of a narrowing.

Progestin: A synthetic form of the female hormone progesterone. Progestin is often used in birth control pills and hormone replacement therapy (HRT).

Pulmonary embolism: Blood clot in the lung.

Pump oxygenator: Commonly called a heart-lung machine, it's used to keep the blood flowing and oxygenated while the heart is stopped during surgery.

Reperfusion therapy: A variety of techniques (including medications, angioplasty, and surgery) that may be used to restore blood flow to areas of the heart damaged by a heart attack.

Resins: Cholesterol-lowering drugs that cause the intestines to absorb less cholesterol from the digestive tract.

Restenosis: The term used when arteries become narrowed again following a procedure to open them.

Risk factors: Traits or lifestyle habits that put one at greater risk for developing certain illnesses or conditions.

Rotational atherectomy: A procedure in which the cardiologist uses a diamond-coated burr to treat conditions such as calcified plaque.

Saphenous vein: The vein that lies just inside the leg. It's often used in bypass surgery.

Saturated fat: The type of fat that comes from animal sources (meat, poultry, fish, egg yolks, dairy products). Solid at room temperature, saturated fat has been associated with the plaque building of atherosclerosis.

Silent ischemia: A temporary shortage of blood and oxygen to the heart that doesn't produce any symptoms.

Single photon emission computed tomography (SPECT): One of the most commonly used nuclear imaging technologies. It involves injecting a radioactive material and then taking images of the chest.

Statins: Drugs often used to reduce cholesterol, statins work directly on the liver to block the manufacture of cholesterol.

Stenosis: Narrowing. In the case of CHD, narrowing of blood vessels.

Stents: Small, fine-mesh tubes that are inserted into arteries to keep them open.

Stroke: Also called a "brain attack," a stroke occurs when one or more blood vessels supplying the brain become blocked, causing the death of brain cells.

Sudden cardiac death (SCD): Sudden and unexpected death caused by the total loss of heart function in someone with or without diagnosed heart disease.

Tachycardia: Abnormally rapid heartbeat.

Thrombolytics: Clot-busting drugs used in the treatment of heart attack.

Total blood cholesterol: A combination of low-density lipoprotein (LDL) and high-density lipoprotein (HDL) cholesterol and triglycerides.

Transmyocardial revascularization (TMR): A technique in which the surgeon drills laser holes into the heart's pumping chamber to relieve chest pain.

Triglycerides: A type of blood fat. Elevated levels of triglycerides are associated with CHD.

Variant angina: Also called Prinzmetal's angina, it's a less common type of chest pain caused when the muscle fibers surrounding the coronary arteries spasm and narrow or completely close off blood vessels that feed the heart.

Vasodilators: Medications that reduce blood pressure by dilating blood vessels.

Vein: One of many vessels that carry blood to the heart.

Ventricles: The lower chambers (one right and one left) of the heart

Venules: Small veins.

Very low-density lipoprotein (VLDL): A type of cholesterol-protein package that contains cholesterol, triglycerides, and protein.

Resources

American Heart Association
National Center
7272 Grandville Avenue
Dallas, TX 75231
800-AHA-USA1 (242-8721)
www.americanheart.org

The American Heart Association's mission is to reduce disability and death from cardiovascular diseases and stroke. It is a not-for-profit, voluntary health organization funded by private contributions. The Web site offers links to message boards, chat rooms, patient guides, caregiver guides, and nutrition and recipe information. The site also features an "Ask the Expert" section.

National Heart, Lung, and Blood Institute (NHLBI)
P.O. Box 30105
Bethesda, MD 20824
301-251-1222
www.nhlbi.nih.gov

The National Heart, Lung, and Blood Institute (NHLBI) provides leadership for a national program in diseases of the heart, blood vessels, lung, and blood; blood resources; and sleep disorders.

The institute plans, conducts, fosters, and supports an integrated and coordinated program of basic research, clinical investigations and trials, observational studies, and demonstration and education projects.

National Institute of Neurological Disorders and Stroke (NINDS)

P.O. Box 5801
Bethesda, MD 20824
800-352-9424
www.ninds.nih.gov

Serving the public and health professionals, the organization offers comprehensive consumer health information, publications, new treatment studies, clinical studies, clinical research training, and research funding.

Pulmonary Hypertension Association

P.O. Box 463
Ambler, PA 19002
800-748-7274
www.phassociation.org

Support and information for patients with pulmonary hypertension, their families, and physicians. Encourages research, promotes awareness, provides resource references. Networking, phone help, pen pals, assistance in starting groups.

Adult Congenital Heart Association (ACHA)

273 Perham Street
West Roxbury, MA 02132
www.achaheart.org

The Adult Congenital Heart Association (ACHA) is a national organization for adults and adolescents with congenital heart disease (CHD). The purpose of the organization is to educate the public, adults with CHD, and the medical community about adult congenital heart issues through the development of forums, newsletters, support groups, and message boards.

American Society of Nuclear Cardiology (ASNC)

9111 Old Georgetown Road
Bethesda, MD 20814
301-493-2360
www.asnc.org

The American Society of Nuclear Cardiology (ASNC) is a professional medical society. The mission of ASNC is to foster optimal delivery of nuclear cardiology services through developing standards of professional education and training, establishing guidelines for the clinical performance of nuclear cardiology, and promoting nuclear cardiology research.

Heart Failure Society of America, Inc.

Court International-Suite 238N
2550 University Avenue West
Saint Paul, MN 55114
651-642-1633
www.hfsa.org

The Heart Failure Society of America, Inc. (HFSA) represents the efforts by heart failure experts from the Americas to provide a forum for all those interested in heart function, heart failure, and congestive heart failure (CHF) research and patient care.

The Mended Hearts, Inc.

7272 Greenville Avenue
Dallas, TX 75231-4596
214-706-1442
www.mendedhearts.org

A nationwide patient support organization comprised of people with heart disease, their families, medical professionals, and other interested persons.

The Coronary Club, Inc.

9500 Euclid Avenue
Mail Code A42
Cleveland, OH 44195
800-478-4255

The Coronary Club, a nonprofit organization, was founded in 1968 to provide patients and their families with information on preventing heart attacks and adjusting to life with a heart condition. Subscribers receive up-to-date reports on coronary care and treatment, diet and exercise, stress management, surgery, and medications. Local chapters hold meetings during which members can exchange experiences and hear speakers.

American Academy of Family Physicians Foundation

11400 Tomahawk Creek Parkway
Leawood, KS 66211-2672
www.familydoctor.org

This organization offers consumer-friendly advise from their book, *Family Health and Medical Guide.* All of the information has been written and reviewed by physicians and patient education professionals at the American Academy of Family Physicians. The information is regularly reviewed and updated.

The American Alliance for Health, Physical Education, Recreation & Dance

1900 Association Drive
Reston, VA 20192-1598
800-213-7193
www.aahperd.org

AAHPERD is an alliance of six national associations, six district associations, and a research consortium all designed to provide members with comprehensive resources, support, and programs to help practitioners improve their skills and so further the health and well-being of the American public.

MEDLINE

www.nih.gov

Produced by the National Library of Medicine, this Web site indexes articles from more than 3,500 medical journals. The service is aimed primarily at scientists and health professionals. MEDLINEPlus is the lay public's version and is found at www.nlm.nih.gov/medlineplus.

NOAH New York Online Access to Health

www.noah-health.org

A consortium of library and medical organizations (the City University of New York, the Metropolitan New York Library Council, the New York Academy of Medicine, and the New York Public Library) that have combined efforts to give consumers free access to many of the best consumer-oriented health materials by respected sources.

Index

64-slice CT scanner, 73

A
abciximab, 88
abdominal obesity, 12
abdominal pain, 41
abnormal heartbeat, 80, 84
    see also arrhythmias
abnormal valve, 76
absorbable sutures, 119
ACE (angiotensin converting
  enzyme) inhibitors, 97, 98
    side effects, 98
ACE inhibitors
    see ACE (angiotensin converting
    enzyme) inhibitors
adult-onset diabetes, 21
    see also diabetes
advance imaging diagnostic tests,
  69–80
aging
    as a risk factor, 12, 14, 31, 50
alcohol use, 27
    excessive, 23, 24, 130
    limiting, 55, 129, 130, 141

with medications, 84
allergic reactions, 76
alpha-blockers, 99, 100
alternative treatment options, 148–
  159
ambulatory ECG, 62
American College of Cardiology, 22,
  158
American Diabetes Association, 128
American Heart Association (AHA),
  4, 11, 17, 46, 48, 52, 125, 130, 153,
  156, 158
American Journal of Cardiology, 157
American Medical Association
  (AMA), 158
amino acid, 24
amlodipine, 86
angina, 9, 33, 34, 62, 103
    changes, 37
    debilitating, 114
    medications, 83, 84
    pattern, 37
    Prinzmetal's, 36
    stable, 35
    as a symptom of heart attack, 41

Index

Index

About the Authors

Barry M. Cohen, M.D., is the medical director of the Cardiac Catheterization Laboratory at the Gagnon Heart Hospital of Morristown, New Jersey. A native of Montreal, he completed his undergraduate studies at McGill University and received his medical degree from the University of Sherbrooke in Canada. Dr. Cohen completed his cardiology fellowship at the Mount Sinai Medical Center in New York, followed by another fellowship in interventional cardiology at the University of California San Diego Medical Center.

Dr. Cohen is a diplomat of the American Board of Internal Medicine and the American Boards of Cardiovascular Disease and Interventional Cardiology. He is a fellow of the American College of Cardiology, the Society of Cardiovascular Angiography and Intervention, and the Royal College of Physician and Surgeons of Canada. He is a past president of the New Jersey Society of Interventional Cardiology and is a practicing clinical cardiologist with Associates in Cardiovascular Disease in Springfield, New Jersey.

Dr. Cohen has published numerous scientific papers and abstracts in interventional cardiology. He pioneered rotational atherectomy used in the treatment of complex calcified coronary arterial blockages, and is an investigator testing new stent designs. He also has an interest in gene and cell therapy research. Dr. Cohen treats stroke victims who have associated heart defects.

Bobbie Hasselbring is an award-winning health writer who has authored or coauthored more than a dozen books on health and psychology. Ms. Hasselbring was a senior editor for *Medical Self-Care*, a national consumer health magazine. She has written for national and regional newspapers and magazines, and for the World Wide Web. She has produced materials for multinational health corporations, pharmaceutical companies, medical publishers, and medical institutions. Ms. Hasselbring has been recognized twice by the American Heart Association for her writing about heart disease and recently won the Rx Club's Excellence in Writing award.

Consumer Health Titles from Addicus Books

Visit our online catalog at www.AddicusBooks.com

Overcoming Postpartum Depression and Anxiety $14.95

A Patient's Guide to Dental Implants $14.95

Prescription Drug Addiction—The Hidden Epidemic $15.95

Prostate Cancer—A Patient's Guide to Treatment $14.95

Simple Changes—The Boomer's Guide
to a Healthier, Happier Life $9.95

A Simple Guide to Thyroid Disorders $14.95

Straight Talk About Breast Cancer—
From Diagnosis to Recovery $15.95

The New Fibromyalgia Remedy $16.95

The Stroke Recovery Book—
A Guide for Patients and Families $14.95

The Surgery Handbook—
A Guide to Understanding Your Operation $14.95

Understanding Lumpectomy—
A Treatment Guide for Breast Cancer $14.95

Understanding Parkinson's Disease—
A Self-Help Guide $14.95

Understanding Peyronie's Disease $16.95

Understanding Your Living Will $12.95

Your Complete Guide to Breast Augmentation
& Body Contouring $21.95

Your Complete Guide to Breast Reduction
& Breast Lifts $21.95

Your Complete Guide to Facial Cosmetic Surgery $19.95

Your Complete Guide to Face-Lifts $21.95

Your Complete Guide to Nose Reshaping $21.95